Affect in Artistic Creativity

Why do painters paint? Obviously, there are numerous possible reasons. They paint to create images for others' enjoyment, to solve visual problems, to convey ideas, and to contribute to a rich artistic tradition. This book argues that there is yet another, crucially important but often overlooked reason.

Painters paint to feel.

They paint because it enables them to experience special feelings, such as being absorbed in creative play and connected to something vitally significant. Painting may even transform the painter's whole sense of being. Thus, painting is not only about producing art, communicating content, and so on, but also about setting up and inhabiting an experiential space wherein highly valued feelings are interactively enabled and supported. This book investigates how and why this happens by combining psychoanalytical theorization on creativity with philosophical thinking on affectivity. It focuses on creative experience itself and illuminates the psychological mechanisms and dynamics that underlie the affects at stake. Painters' own descriptions of how they feel at work are used throughout to give an accurate, true-to-life portrayal of the experience of painting.

The strength of the book lies in its open-minded yet critical integration of contemporary psychoanalytic and philosophical thinking, and in its truthfulness to painters' experiential descriptions of the painterly process. On the whole, it enriches our understanding of artistic creativity and sheds more light on how and why we come to feel the things we do. As such, the book will appeal to philosophers, psychoanalysts, and art researchers alike.

Jussi A. Saarinen, PhD, is a psychologist and postdoctoral researcher in philosophy at the University of Jyväskylä, Finland. His interests lie in psychoanalytical aesthetics and philosophy of emotion, and he has published on these topics in journals including *The International Journal of Psychoanalysis*, *The Journal of Aesthetics and Art Criticism*, and *Phenomenology and the Cognitive Sciences*.

Art, Creativity, and Psychonalysis Book Series

Series Editor

George Hagman, LSCW

The *Art, Creativity, and Psychoanalysis* book series seeks to highlight original, cutting edge studies of the relationship between psychoanalysis and the world of art and the psychology of artists, with subject matter including the psychobiography of artists, the creative process, the psychology of aesthetic experience, as well as the aesthetic, creative and artistic aspects of psychoanalysis and psychoanalytic psychotherapy. *Art, Creativity, and Psychoanalysis* promotes a vision of psychoanalysis as a creative art, the clinical effectiveness of which can be enhanced when we better understand and utilize artistic and creative processes at its core.

The series welcomes proposals from psychoanalytic therapists from all professional groups and theoretical models, as well as artists, art historians and art critics informed by a psychoanalytic perspective.

Psychoanalysis, Intersubjective Writing, and a Postmaterialist Model of Mind
I Woke Up Dead
Dan Gilhooley, Frank Toich

Poetry and Psychoanalysis
The Opening of the Field
David Shaddock

Affect in Artistic Creativity
Painting to Feel
Jussi A. Saarinen

For a full list of all titles in the series, please visit the Routledge website at: https://www.routledge.com/ACAPBS.

Affect in Artistic Creativity

Painting to Feel

Jussi A. Saarinen

Routledge
Taylor & Francis Group
LONDON AND NEW YORK

First published 2021
by Routledge
2 Park Square, Milton Park, Abingdon, Oxon OX14 4RN

and by Routledge
52 Vanderbilt Avenue, New York, NY 10017

Routledge is an imprint of the Taylor & Francis Group, an informa business

British Library Cataloguing-in-Publication Data
A catalogue record for this book is available from the British Library

Library of Congress Cataloging-in-Publication Data
A catalog record for this book has been requested

ISBN: 978-0-367-52249-0 (hbk)
ISBN: 978-0-367-52247-6 (pbk)
ISBN: 978-1-003-05716-1 (ebk)

Typeset in Times New Roman
by Apex CoVantage, LLC

The following chapters of the book build on previously published texts.

Chapter 2, "Painting as affective scaffolding", builds on:

- Saarinen, J. A. (2019). Paintings as solid affective scaffolds. *Journal of Aesthetics and Art Criticism*, 77 (1), 67–77.

Chapter 5, "Oceanic feeling", builds on:

- Saarinen, J. A. (2015). The concept of the oceanic feeling in artistic creativity and in the analysis of visual artworks. *Journal of Aesthetic Education*, 49 (3), 15–31; and
- Saarinen, J. A. (2015). *A Conceptual Analysis of the Oceanic Feeling – With a Special Note on Painterly Aesthetics*. Jyväskylä: *Jyväskylä Studies in Education, Psychology and Social Research*.

Chapter 7, "Painting and existential feeling", builds on:

- Saarinen, J. A. (2014). The oceanic feeling in painterly creativity. *Contemporary Aesthetics*, vol. 12. www.contempaesthetics.org; and
- Saarinen, J. A. (2018). A critical examination of existential feeling. *Phenomenology and the Cognitive Sciences*, 17 (2), 363–374.

Contents

Foreword

George Hagman, LCSW

Several years ago, when we were developing the plan for the *Art, Creativity, and Psychoanalysis* book series, it was my hope to create a publishing platform for new authors, researchers, and clinicians from various disciplines and schools of thought, hailing from all over the world. Then I received an email from Dr. Jussi Saarinen, a psychologist and postdoctoral researcher in philosophy in Finland. I found that Jussi shares my passion for art and the psychology of the artists and the creative process. Similar to me, his interests lie in psychoanalytic aesthetics and the role of emotion in art. Jussi has published on these topics in journals including *The International Journal of Psychoanalysis*, *The Journal of Aesthetics and Art Criticism*, and *Phenomenology and the Cognitive Sciences*. He has also painted and drawn for many years, and at one point in time seriously considered becoming a professional artist. Over the past few years, Jussi and I have exchanged many emails, and I have followed his career from the United States with the aid of the internet. Jussi's work focuses on the place of affect in art and artistic creativity (interestingly, including the 'oceanic feeling', which has in recent years been neglected by psychoanalysis), existential feelings, object relations theory, and the self – all from the viewpoint of a researcher attempting to understand the mysteries of art. With time, Jussi's list of publications has grown in volume, quality, and depth of knowledge and insight, and it has now become evident that he has created a body of work that is ready to be brought together in a monograph, documenting in full his exciting exploration of the mind of the artist. Now I am pleased to publish Jussi's first book as part of the *Art, Creativity, and Psychoanalysis* book series. Being able to give Jussi this opportunity not only to organize his thoughts into a sustained and complete volume, but also to be able to make his work known to the academic and psychoanalytic communities, gives me a great deal of satisfaction. I guarantee that all of you, upon reading Jussi's book, *Affect in Artistic Creativity: Painting to Feel*, will gain new insights into why artists paint, what drives them on despite the difficult challenges they face, and what the nature is of that special affective passion which draws them to color and form as they search for an experience which will scaffold the self, and perhaps even accomplish a small triumph over mortality.

Preface

Although this book has been written in just over a year, it brings together ideas that have taken shape over the past decade or so. In late 2008, I launched into a doctoral dissertation that dealt with so-called oceanic feelings of self-boundary dissolution and unity. My interest in the topic arose mainly from artists' – and especially painters' – descriptions of merging with the works they were creating. With an amateur background in painting, I had even experienced hints and whispers of such feelings myself. To gain a better grasp of this intriguing yet surprisingly widespread phenomenon, I turned to psychoanalytical research into mysticism and creativity, and to contemporary philosophical discussions about feelings, emotions, and moods. Through these theoretical perspectives, I began to see both the practice of painting and the nature of our affective lives in an altogether novel light. Crucially, I realized that painting involved various *affective objectives* that had not, to my knowledge, been examined sufficiently in existing investigations into artistic creativity. In short, I came to understand that painters paint in order to feel things. The present book has grown out of this (seemingly) simple observation.

Numerous people have helped make this book a reality, and to them I owe my deepest gratitude. Having said that, I cannot possibly name all the individuals and groups who have, over the last ten years, helped me develop its main themes. I must therefore limit my acknowledgments to those who have been involved in the formation of this book during the last few years. To begin, were it not for George Hagman, the editor of the *Art, Creativity, and Psychoanalysis* series at Routledge, the book would not have come into being at all. I am immensely grateful for his suggestion to gather my thoughts on painting into a full-length study and for offering to include it in this newly launched series, and for taking the time to review it carefully.

Throughout my work, I have been very fortunate to receive comments, insights, and support from inspiring people across various disciplines. First of all, I want to express my gratitude to fellow members of the multidisciplinary Experiential Demarcation research group: Joona Taipale, Sanna Tirkkonen, Heidi Fast, Petra Nyman-Salonen, and Tiia-Mari Hovila. Thank you for reading and commenting on several unfinished chapters of the book. Your shrewd and encouraging feedback has been invaluable this past year. I especially wish to thank Joona for many stimulating conversations about just about every topic contained in this book, and for giving me the opportunity to dedicate myself to writing it full time. This kind of commitment would not have been possible without proper financial resources, either. I thus owe the Kone Foundation a massive debt of gratitude for funding the Experiential Demarcation Project generously for four full years.

I am greatly indebted to Giovanna Colombetti, Joel Krueger, and Matthew Ratcliffe, without whose work this study would not have the philosophical basis that it does. Each has been willing to discuss their ideas on affectivity with open and critical minds – a philosophical virtue I truly admire. Thanks also to Tom Roberts for the positive feedback given in Tallinn. As for the psychoanalytical side of the story, I am grateful to Henrik Enckell for organizing the meetings of the Psychoanalytical Research Consortium in Helsinki, where I have had the opportunity to discuss oceanic feelings and creativity with a group of knowledgeable psychoanalysts and psychoanalytical researchers. Päivi Aho-Mustonen, in turn, has kindly invited me to share my thoughts on painting with psychoanalysts in my hometown of Jyväskylä. I would also like to thank psychoanalyst and visual artist Patricia Townsend for making her way to Finland to discuss her research on creative states of mind. Her work has been indispensable to my own study. Luckily, I have had the opportunity to talk with other professional artists about their work, as well. I am particularly grateful to Olli Piippo for allowing me to probe into his personal painterly practices. His generous observations on the affective aspects of the creative process have given me much food for thought. I would also like to thank Anna-Leena Vilhunen for inviting me to her studio to talk about art and art-making. It is a special privilege to be allowed into the space where the magic happens.

Finally, my greatest gratitude is reserved for my partner, Nina Reiman, whose support has been unwavering during the entire intensive process of writing this book. Not only has she engaged in enlightening conversations about key themes of the book and given me the necessary room to write, but she has also been willing to help resolve whatever formal and theoretical quandaries I have found myself in.

All of the chapters in this book have been written exclusively for the present study and are thus intended to constitute a cohesive and coherent whole. However, some of the chapters do rework and elaborate on ideas and arguments that have been previously published. Chapter 2 builds on "Paintings as Solid Affective Scaffolds", published in 2019 in the *Journal of Aesthetics and Art Criticism*, 77 (1), 67–77, and on "What Can the Concept of Affective Scaffolding Do for Us", forthcoming in *Philosophical Psychology*. Chapter 5, in turn, combines and reworks ideas from the following two texts: "The Concept of the Oceanic Feeling in Artistic Creativity and in the Analysis of Visual Artworks", published in 2015 in *Journal of Aesthetic Education*, 49 (3), 15–31, and the "Introduction" to my PhD thesis, *A Conceptual Analysis of the Oceanic Feeling – With a Special Note on Painterly Aesthetics*, published by *Jyväskylä Studies in Education, Psychology and Social Research* in 2015. Finally, Chapter 7 redevelops ideas expressed in "The Oceanic Feeling in Painterly Creativity", published online in 2014 in *Contemporary Aesthetics*, vol. 12, and "A Critical Examination of Existential Feeling", published in 2018 in *Phenomenology and the Cognitive Sciences*, 17 (2), 363–374. The peer reviews and editorial advice I have received from these journals have considerably increased the cogency of the argument put forward in this study.

Chapter 1

Framing the issue

Why do painters paint? Of course, there are numerous possible reasons: to produce artworks for others' enjoyment, to solve visual problems, to experiment with a medium, to communicate personal ideas, and to contribute to a longstanding artistic tradition, to name just a few of the most obvious incentives. In this book I argue that there is yet another, critically important but often overlooked reason.

Painters paint *to feel*.

They paint because it conjures a sense of intimacy, or makes them feel stimulated and challenged, or absorbed by something mysterious and meaningful. It makes them feel alive and creative and liberated from the constraints of life. Painters may also paint in order to deal with loss – to grieve. It makes them feel sheltered. At home.

Safe.

And sound.

Painting is thus an activity that enables various desirable and highly valued affective states. In this study, I explore *how* and *why* this is so. To support and illustrate my ideas, I also analyze several special feelings that are evoked by painting in the proposed manner. On the whole, this means that I consider paintings – or, more accurately, paintings-*in-progress* – as means to affective ends rather than as objects of aesthetic evaluation or psychobiographical interpretation. I have next to nothing to say about individual painters' lives or the reception of their paintings. Nor do I dig deep into the various ideological, historical, and cultural factors that influence painters' artistic self-conceptions and dispositions. Although such factors contribute greatly to the experience of painting, I focus first and foremost on creative *experience itself* and on the psychological mechanisms and dynamics that underlie the affects at stake. To achieve a truthful picture of the experience of painting, I substantiate my account throughout with painters' own descriptions of how they feel while they work, as documented in interviews, biographies and autobiographies, artist's monographs, exhibition texts, and so forth.

On the whole, the proposed view will be developed by integrating philosophical thinking on affectivity with psychoanalytical theorization on creativity. But why these two approaches? Can they provide appropriate conceptual tools for investigating the matter, and do they make a good mutual fit? Much philosophical research on creativity has tended to foreground cognition at the expense of affect, for instance by prioritizing problem solving, imagination, and divergent thinking over the 'feel' of creative activity. To give just one example, a recent collection of essays on the philosophy of creativity mentions 'affect' and 'emotion' a mere handful of times, and even then, as more or less subsidiary phenomena to cognition (see Paul & Kaufman, 2014). This is not to deny the merits of these contributions but to highlight their priorities in studying the phenomenon.

There is more to the story, though, for philosophers have clearly had something to say about the role of emotions and feelings in artistic creativity as well. One need only look at the question of *expression* in the field of aesthetics to see that this is the case (see, e.g., Collingwood, 1938/1969; Nahm, 1955; Khatchadourian, 1965; Graham, 2005; Matravers, 2010; Wiltsher, 2017). In its narrowest form, the expressionist theory of art holds that artistic work is, or at least involves, an expression of the artist's own feelings and emotions, be they conscious or unconscious. A broader form of the theory allows that artworks can express – or be expressive *of* – ideas and feelings more generally, apart from whatever their makers think and feel. Whether that or the other is the case has been a heated topic of debate for decades now.

That being said, I intend to sidestep the issue of expression as far as possible, for two main reasons. First, I do not want to get mired in semantic disputes over what it means 'to express an emotion' or what 'the expression of feeling in art' would necessitate. Indeed, owing to its ambiguity, I generally avoid using the term 'expression' altogether. Second, and more importantly, the focal point of this study lies elsewhere – that is, in the *evocation* rather than the expression of affect. Simply put, I am primarily interested in the affective *effects* of painting: how it permits the painter to feel things that would otherwise be difficult if not impossible to feel. In short, painters probably paint because they feel, but I highlight the feelings they feel because they paint.

So where, then, do I suggest we turn for suitable philosophical insight into the painterly pursuit of affect? Contemporary philosophers of mind have used the concepts of *scaffolding* and *niche construction* to anatomize how our active engagements with the world influence our feeling, thinking, and doing. Put broadly, 'scaffolding' designates the various ways in which environmental resources – such as things, other people, physical spaces, etc. – are used to elicit, regulate, and augment our affects, cognitions, and actions (see Colombetti & Krueger, 2015; Sterelny, 2010; Sutton, 2016). The term 'niche construction' has been applied similarly to detail the various processes whereby we manipulate our material, social, epistemic, and cultural landscapes to support and enhance our psychological and experiential capabilities (see Clark, 2006; Sterelny, 2010; Sutton, Harris, Keil, & Barnier, 2010). Integrating the key points of these conceptualizations amounts to the following premise: we build niches to scaffold our minds. It is this basic idea that I apply to painting in the present study. Viewed in this light, painting involves setting up a creative niche in which paintings-in-progress scaffold the artist's ongoing emotions, moods, and other affective states.

I maintain that 'niche construction' and 'affective scaffolding' are particularly useful in analyzing the *formal* and *structural* aspects of artists' affect-inducing exchanges with their paintings. However, these concepts can only take us so far in grasping the affective *dynamics* of the creative process. For one thing, they cannot really shed much light on why certain affective states become individually important and desirable in painting. Nor do they explain how the activity of painting develops into a crucial resource for such feelings in the first place. In sum, what is lacking from the given philosophical approach is an in-depth psychological understanding of what *drives* our scaffolding interactions and how these interactions incorporate lengthy *personal histories* of feeling. Hence, we need a complementary account of why painters come to seek certain feelings in relation to their artwork, and how paintings in turn come to function as invaluable scaffolds for such feelings.

This is where psychoanalysis makes a timely entry into the discussion. Psychoanalytical research incorporates a long tradition of studying the developmental roots and unconscious dynamics of artistic creation. Moreover, in fleshing out these aspects of creativity, psychoanalytical theoreticians have often provided thorough observations concerning the actual *experience* of art-making. In some cases, the thinkers in question have been artists themselves; in others, they have interviewed or even taught artists. Psychoanalysis thus constitutes an incomparably abundant reservoir of theoretical and experiential knowledge on the creative mind and the artistic process.

Drawing mainly from so-called relationally oriented psychoanalytical thinking, and especially from the work of one of its most prominent figures, D. W. Winnicott, I maintain that painting is a reciprocal activity conditioned by early interactions with others, and that it is accordingly motivated and organized by primal, relationally established affective concerns, such as the need to achieve meaningful and vital contacts with one's surroundings. From this point of view, painting is seen as a creative form of object-relating that is deeply rooted in the earliest interactions between the infant and the caretaking environment. This also means that painters come to their here-and-now engagements with paintings from a lengthy and complexly patterned background of personal affective scaffoldings. Simply put, individual developmental history significantly influences what painters seek to feel via painting, and how they come to achieve this.

At this point, it is worth mentioning that most psychoanalytical models of artistic creativity follow some variant of the previously mentioned expressionist approach to art. Typically, these models presuppose that the artist projects elements of inchoate affective experience into the developing artwork, in and through which these elements are then shaped into and expressed in novel form, and finally reintegrated back into the artist's enhanced sense of self. To reiterate, I do not intend to delve into the expressive side of creation, although I do reflect on it when necessary, especially when the scaffolded affect under scrutiny can be made intelligible only in relation to the articulation and formalization of the artist's experience. Overall, however, I shift the spotlight on to the enablement and evocation of affects which cannot be said to exist, even formlessly, prior to the painterly endeavor, and which are essentially made possible and supported by the activity of painting itself. Simply put, I aim to analyze the co-constitution of novel affects through painter–painting interaction. This entails that, by way of painting, artists seek to experience feelings that are not in any sense latent and therefore 'merely waiting' to be articulated and expressed. I take my lead here from psychoanalyst George Hagman, who also suggests a "new perspective on creativity, in which the *artist actively seeks to bring about an experience* to confirm and/or repair his or her sense of self" (Hagman, 2005, p. 68, my italics). To be clear, the advocated approach is by no means incompatible with expressionist theories of art; however, fleshing out and arguing for the latter falls beyond the scope of the present study.

All in all, then, by combining key contributions from both philosophy and psychoanalysis, this study seeks to open up new perspectives on affectivity in painting. This will be done without subordinating either discipline to the other. The two are applied as complementary and equally important building blocks in the proposed argument. First, philosophy is used to develop a cogent account of how the act of painting, as a creative interaction with an environmental resource, enables the painter to attain and sustain desirable feelings. Psychoanalysis, in turn, is used to specify the developmental, dynamic, and relational underpinnings of these affective processes; it thus provides the examination with a depth and ontogenetic awareness missing from the philosophical approach. Overall, I would like to think that the relevance and strength of this study lies precisely in its open-minded yet critical integration of (mostly contemporary) psychoanalytic and philosophical thinking, and in its truthfulness to painters' first-person experiential descriptions of painting.

To reiterate, my main thesis is that painting is not *only* about producing art, conveying feelings and ideas, and so on, but also about setting up and inhabiting a niche in which certain highly valued affects are interactively enabled, supported, and regulated. I would also like to point out that the feelings discussed in this study are not just any old feelings, so to speak. Rather, they pertain to profound and deeply ingrained human concerns over subjective and objective reality, meaningful and vital living, and the boundaries between self, others, and the world. That is to say, some of the most intense and valued feelings enabled by painting – such as the feelings of fluidity, unity, resonance, and aliveness – bear directly on how we 'find ourselves in the world'. Painters pursue the mentioned kinds of affects via painting because they galvanize, enrich, and (re)structure their overall sense of being. This means that painting and painterly affectivity carry considerable *existential import* – a fact that I will consistently underline and elaborate on throughout this study.

Finally, with all this talk about feelings, emotions, and affects, the term 'affectivity' calls for a bit more clarification. What, exactly, does it refer to? Needless to say, there are numerous competing accounts, taxonomies, and theories out there. I will not wade into this debate here. Instead, I will briefly discuss one alternative for identifying and distinguishing between different phenomena belonging to the so-called "affective realm" (Ben-Ze'ev, 1997). This will serve to illustrate the multifaceted nature of affectivity and, more importantly, to elucidate how I generally conceive of it in this study.

There are two criteria that are particularly apposite to the given classificatory task: (1) the *intentionality*, and (2) the *actuality vs. potentiality* of the state under consideration (Ben-Ze'ev, 1997, pp. 248–249; see also Goldie, 2000; Colombetti & Roberts, 2015). Here, 'intentionality' means that mental states are *about* or *directed towards* some object or the other, be it specific (such as another person) or diffuse (such as the world in general). Affective states, too, are intentional, but to add to that, they are states that disclose their intentional objects on a positive–negative continuum. In short, they are *evaluative* intentional states. For example, the painter's satisfaction with her work involves a positive evaluation of the intentional object of her feeling, namely, the painting. However, mere evaluation does not suffice for a state to be affective: the painter may judge her work to be satisfactory without actually feeling so. Indeed, a combination of the evaluative intentional dimension with a significant *feeling dimension* distinguishes affective states from non-affective ones (Ben-Ze'ev, 1997, p. 248). As for the second criterion, mental states can generally be said to be either *occurrent* or *dispositional*. For example, at a certain moment the painter may feel her painting to be going down the drain; indeed, she might feel downright frustrated and dispirited. At the same time, she may be fundamentally predisposed to feel that her artistic efforts will, on the whole, be successful. The painter thus has a basic inclination to feel optimistic about her work despite being momentarily dejected.

By charting possible variations in (1) the intentionality of the evaluative stand and (2) the actuality/potentiality of the feeling dimension, we arrive at four basic types of affective phenomena (Ben-Ze'ev, 1997, p. 249). *Emotions* are occurrent states of feeling that take on relatively specific intentional objects. For example, one may feel proud of a personal achievement or disappointed at being let down by a friend. *Moods*, like emotions, are occurrent states of feeling, but involve more diffuse intentionality. One may, for instance, feel angry at nothing in particular and everything in general – at the whole world, as it were. Emotions and moods tend to occur episodically, with emotions typically lasting from minutes to hours and moods from hours and days to weeks, and perhaps even months. *Sentiments*, in turn, can be seen as dispositional states that concern specific intentional objects. An example of this would be enduring love for one's partner. In this case, the love can be said to 'be there' even when it is not explicitly manifest in the occurrent emotion felt towards the other. Finally, *affective traits* are dispositional states that have general intentionality. In this category we find traits such as enviousness, which may predispose the individual to feel jealous of any number of things, and which can even last for an entire lifetime. In sum, on this view the affective realm consists of two occurrent states, emotions and moods, and of two dispositional states, sentiments and affective traits.

There is certainly more to affectivity than the presented classification permits. For instance, it has been posited that, in addition to emotions and moods, we experience atmospheric feelings, feelings of being alive, and vitality affects, none of which fall neatly into the stated categories (see Fuchs, 2013; Ratcliffe, 2008; Stern, 1985, respectively). Indeed, in the final chapter of this book, I also discuss a special class of feeling that is not properly recognized by the aforementioned taxonomical approach. That being said, my focus is predominantly on *occurrent* affective states. Moreover, seeing as we *feel* emotions, moods, atmospheric feelings, and other such affects, I will in practice subsume all of these felt affects under the general term of *feelings*. I do so because identifying the specific class of affect that is being scaffolded by painting is not particularly relevant for the main argument of the study. Instead of burdening the reader with taxonomical concerns and technicalities, I concentrate on the affective *experiences* themselves – that is, on how they feel and what they mean for the artist.

Having introduced the objectives and theoretical framework of this book, I will now outline its overall structure and contents, chapter by chapter. In different ways, the chapters support and advance the main claim of the study – that painters paint to feel. It is also worth noting that each chapter foregrounds two or three theoreticians whose thoughts I consider particularly pertinent to the theoretical issues and affective states under examination, and with whom I thus converse to develop my own account. Many of these thinkers – especially those working within the relational framework – share several key ideas about the nature, development, and dynamics of artistic creativity. Again, whenever I discuss these ideas in the upcoming chapters, I draw selectively from a couple of theoreticians at a time rather than accommodating everyone's contributions all at once. This entails that various closely connected thoughts from various different thinkers will be spread out evenly across the entire book. This will allow me to develop and diversify the main themes of the study gradually and cumulatively. Inevitably, this will also lead to some overlapping content, and it is on such occasions that I ask the reader for patience.

So, in Chapter 2, I advance the overall philosophical framework of the study. I first spell out how the concepts of *affective scaffolding* and *niche construction* contribute to our understanding of the 'life of the mind'. I then move on to identify various *dimensions* along which the scaffolded mind can vary. More specifically, I examine affective scaffolding – both in general and in relation to painting – with respect to elemental structure, temporality, reciprocality, individuality and collectivity, trust, individualization and entrenchment, and intent. This analysis serves two purposes. First, it demonstrates that scaffolding interactions come in a wide variety of forms, and second, it serves to delimit the scope of my analyses of the special affects scaffolded by painting (presented in Chapters 4–6). Based on the multidimensional model, I fix the spotlight solely on the kind of painterly interaction that is constituted by *synchronic reciprocality* between an *active individual agent* and a resource that is *sufficiently distinct* and *reliably efficacious* with regard to the agent's desired affects. To conclude, I reflect on some of the limitations of the given philosophical perspective and, based on this, motivate the need for a complementary approach to affective scaffolding in painting. Basically, I suggest that what is required is a better understanding of the ontogenetic underpinnings of painterly interaction, and also of the unconsciously structured needs and concerns that motivate this interaction.

Thus, in Chapter 3, I turn to psychoanalytical theorization, and Winnicott's thinking in particular, to fill in these gaps. My basic premise is that early development shapes later creative activity in various significant ways. To elaborate on this idea, I first discuss how individuals are born into caretaking niches which, from the start, provide developmentally crucial affective scaffoldings. More specifically, I examine how early infant–caregiver interactions instill in the baby the basic capacity and confidence to *engage creatively* with the world. From this starting point the creative attitude gradually extends and diversifies to encompass a variety of external objects, including works of art. Moreover, I argue that at this early stage several *core concerns* pertaining to one's being are set into motion – concerns which inevitably, yet mostly unconsciously, continue to bear upon adult experience and behavior. I introduce four such existential concerns, namely, how to relate *subjective* and *objective* realities; how to demarcate between *me* and *not-me*; how to cope with *separation* and the associated need for meaningful *connection* with others; and how to achieve and strengthen the sense of being *fully alive*. Overall, I submit that painting enables the artist to attend to and play with these interrelated concerns creatively. I also suggest that many of the feelings most valued by painters are inextricably linked to how this existential play unfolds in the painterly process. To illustrate these points, in Chapters 4–6 I investigate three special feelings scaffolded by painting, each of which holds considerable existential import for the painter.

In Chapter 4, I discuss the first of these feelings, namely, the peculiar feeling of one's paintings *being alive*. I submit that there are two main variations of this vitalistic experience. First, paintings can be experienced simply as *organic* things – that is, as things that possess certain attributes of living matter, such as the ability to grow and to develop. Second, paintings may additionally be experienced as *agentive* organic things, for instance, as responsive and autonomous contributors to the creative process. To elaborate on this observation, I identify three types of factors that contribute to the aliveness of paintings. First, I discuss the importance of *cultural* and *discursive* factors. In other words, I consider the ways in which extant conceptions of artistic creativity support animistic notions of painting and thus foster the experience of paintings as living and agentive beings. Following this, I shift to the *psychological* and *developmental* factors that underlie the given feelings. I focus specifically on artists' vitalistic fantasies and expectations, and examine how these underlying, mostly unconscious factors are rooted in early dyadic interaction. Third, I call attention to some of the *material* and *metamorphic* factors that account for feelings of aliveness. I discuss the vitality-inducing tactile and visual qualities of paint itself and, along with this, illuminate how the transformation of paintings during the creative process makes them more liable to be experienced as living things. Finally, I underline that the aliveness of one's paintings also enables *oneself* to feel more alive and connected. In this manner, the given feelings satisfy core existential strivings for vitalizing and enriching contacts with the surrounding world.

In Chapter 5, I examine so-called *oceanic feelings* in painting. These are, in short, feelings of self-boundary dissolution and fusion with one's paintings-in-progress. In the first part of the chapter, I elaborate on the experiential features, generative mechanisms, and potential value of oceanic feelings in light of ongoing theoretical debates on the topic. Along with this, I maintain that dissolution and fusion experiences are inextricably bound up with the core existential concerns of, for example, intermixing subjective and objective reality and of demarcating between self and not-self. In the second part of the chapter, I analyze oceanic feelings specifically in the context of painterly creativity. I argue that oceanic experience may support and enhance painting in two crucial ways. On the one hand, it incorporates a mode of *undifferentiated perception* that can be used to manage the complexity of artistic creativity and to advance novel symbol formation. Second, oceanic feelings typically come with various positive *secondary affects* that may serve to protect, vitalize, and guide the creative process. For these reasons, many painters come to regard oceanic states as highly valuable to their creative work.

In Chapter 6, I analyze the climactic feeling of getting one's painting to work or, simply, of *getting it right*. My guiding premise is that, via painting, painters aim to articulate elements of their own experience, where 'experience' is to be understood as broadly possible. Accordingly, I suggest that feelings of correctness depend on how successfully these experiential elements are formalized in the developing work. Moreover, I maintain that we learn to articulate elements of our inchoate experience in and through our earliest interactions with others. Crucially, when our experiential states are reflected and corroborated through these primary exchanges, we undergo rudimentary feelings of fittingness, harmony, and resonance. This, I argue, instills in us the permanent desire to engage with objects that feel right, and that make *us* feel right, too. All in all, then, I propose that feelings of getting it right have a *dual structure*. On the one hand, they depend on and become intelligible in relation to the specific experiential elements that are being worked on in the painting. This aspect of correctness hinges on how well the underlying aim of formalizing certain aspects of one's experiential world is fulfilled by the created work. On the other hand, feelings of rightness may be connected to one's existence in a more comprehensive manner. This side of the feeling depends on having one's overall sense of being reflected back to oneself in ideal form by the painting. In essence, the need to 'get it right' thus involves the perpetual existential concerns of being fully alive and meaningfully connected with one's surroundings.

Finally, in Chapter 7, I focus exclusively on the idea that painting not only scaffolds various episodic feelings but also supports the modification and sustenance of the artist's overall, affectively constituted orientation to the world. In short, I argue that painting can serve to scaffold the artist's fundamental *feelings of being*. To support this claim, I first provide a case study of psychoanalyst Marion Milner's experimentation with painting. Then, to tease out the existential reverberations of her painterly project, I inspect it from the viewpoint of philosopher Matthew Ratcliffe's theory of so-called existential feelings. After discussing how existential feelings constitute a changeable background sense of belonging to and relating to the world as a whole, I suggest that Milner's creative progression can be understood both as temporary shifts in existential feeling and as the gradual consolidation of a more permanent existential orientation. Based on this analysis, I conclude that existential feeling can become one of the main *objects* of artistic creativity, that is, *that which is worked on* in painting. This means that, through painting, artists can tap into and reorganize their experiential worlds vis-à-vis self-other demarcation, separateness, connectedness, vitality, and so on. In sum, my aim is to show that painting, and especially a long-term commitment to painting, can significantly reconfigure how one 'finds oneself in the world'.

Before proceeding on to the subject matter proper, I want to say a few final words about the overall aims and range of this study. In addition to the previously stated, relatively specific contributions, the study has two overarching and complementary objectives. The first is to argue for the centrality of affectivity in painting more generally and, in doing so, to enrich both psychoanalytical and philosophical theorization on artistic creativity. Second, through the systematic exposition of scaffolded affect in painting, the study aims to increase and diversify our understanding of the overall nature of affective experiencing – of how and why we normally come to feel the things we do.

Without question, this study also has its limitations. Seeing as the proposed account is restricted to a dyadically structured and reciprocally unfolding type of painting which, moreover, accentuates the actions and experiences of the individual artist, it inevitably leaves out various other types of painterly praxes. That is to say, given that painters paint in a wide variety of ways and with numerous different objectives, I do not think that *all* painting necessarily involves the specified kind of affective scaffolding. Nor, indeed, do I maintain that it *should*. Thus, I avoid making any universal or normative claims about what painting is and what it should endeavor to achieve. At the same time, I maintain that many painters *do*, in fact, relate to their works and experience the creative process in ways portrayed in this study. My more moderate position is therefore that under certain conditions painting *can* function as a significant affective scaffold to painters, and that under these conditions it may also engender the specified, highly valued feelings.

Finally, I do not want to give the impression that painting necessarily involves intense feelings all the time or even most of the time. On the contrary, for most painters, painting inevitably includes considerable stretches of low-key feeling, such as mild enthusiasm or weariness, and moments of plain old dullness and tedium, to boot. The frequency and intensity of any given feeling will depend on numerous different things, including the artist's temperament, affective dispositions, methods of working, and artistic aims, and on how the work is progressing and developing. Ultimately, on the occasions that painting *does* succeed in scaffolding relatively strong feelings of vitality, fusion, resonance, and the like, the potential existential impact of these feelings will not necessarily be simple and direct. It would be overly schematic to argue, for instance, that each feeling maps neatly on to one existential concern only. Case in point, the oceanic feeling is not only bound up with concerns about demarcating between self and not-self but also about bringing together subjective and objective realities, of coping with separation and the need for meaningful connections, and of achieving a vital sense of being. What's more, instead of effecting great changes immediately, the given feelings may exert their influence on the artist's overall existential orientation on an extended timescale, gradually and subtly. In sum, scaffolded affect may manifest in episodic and occasionally quite impassioned bursts, but it may also be a rather prolonged, slow-burn affair. It is, in short, a multiform and complex phenomenon.

Chapter 2

Painting as affective scaffolding

We engage with our surroundings continuously in order to influence how we feel. We rely on highly sophisticated streaming services for entertainment and pleasure, forge therapeutic alliances to transform our emotional dispositions, and spend hours playing games – just for the sheer contentment of it. Such active manipulation of the environment for affective effects has been designated in recent philosophy of mind as *affective scaffolding*. Here 'scaffolding' quite literally means that our affective states are supported by environmental resources such as material objects, other people, and physical spaces. As such, the concept of scaffolding enables us to investigate in detail how our feelings are embedded in and dependent on the contexts in which they occur.

The idea of scaffolding also encourages us to look anew at how feelings figure in the process of painting. For most artists, painting is not just something that they do, but a fundamental aspect of their very being. Given such weighty personal investment and import, it is only natural that the creative process will involve a host of positive, negative, and mixed feelings. Indeed, if painting truly *matters*, the artist is bound to feel frustrated in the face of seemingly insoluble problems, energized by fortuitous accidents on the canvas, and delighted by major advances in the work – to name just a few of many painting-induced feelings. In short, artistic creativity is an affectively charged affair. However, whereas most discussion has focused on the *expression* of feeling in and through art, considerably less has been said about artists' active pursuit and attainment of various affective states by way of the creative process. I will develop the latter notion by arguing that, for many painters, painting is not only or necessarily about giving form to personal experience, about communicating certain contents, or even about producing finished works for display. It is equally about the creation of a personal niche in which certain desirable and otherwise elusive feelings are enabled, realized, and valued. Simply put, painters *paint to feel.*

In this chapter, I will expound on this key claim as follows. I first summarize how the theories of *situated mind* and *niche construction* contribute to the concept of affective scaffolding. I also clarify the general manner in which I use the concept to appreciate the significance of affect in painting. I then move on to identify various *dimensions* along which scaffolding can vary and, conjointly, apply these dimensions to painting to illuminate its functioning as an affective scaffold. I highlight certain dimensional features in order to delineate the scope of my analysis in later chapters and to draw attention to the ways in which paintings differ from other forms of affective scaffolding. To conclude, I discuss some of the limitations of the account I am proposing and, based on this, motivate the need for a complementary developmental approach to painterly affectivity. The latter will be introduced and integrated with the notion of scaffolding in the next chapter.

Situatedness, niche construction, and affective scaffolding

The notion of scaffolding is premised on the mind's *situatedness* (see, e.g., Griffiths & Scarantino, 2009; Stephan, Walter, & Wilutzky, 2014; Wilson & Clark, 2009). This means that our mental processes are fundamentally codetermined by the circumstances and environmental contexts in which they occur, and therefore cannot be explained solely in terms of what takes place physiologically in our brains or, more broadly, within our individual organismic boundaries. The technical term 'scaffolding' has accordingly been adopted to designate the various ways in which external environmental elements are used to support, regulate, augment, and enhance our cognitions, affects, and mental functioning (see, e.g., Clark, 1997; Colombetti, 2017b; Colombetti & Krueger, 2015; Sterelny, 2010; Sutton, 2016). Overall, in accounting for the life of the mind, the situated approach underscores continuous agent–environment interaction. The key ramification of this idea is that scaffolds are structured and employed through our *active engagements* with the world.

Some philosophical proponents of the scaffolded mind have also drawn on the biological theory of *niche construction* to develop and defend their views. Put broadly, niche construction refers to activities and processes whereby organisms modify their selective environments in ways that affect their own behavior and evolutionary fitness, and typically those of future generations and other species as well (Odling-Smee, Laland, & Feldman, 2003; Laland, Matthews, & Feldman, 2016). For example, earthworms alter the structure and chemistry of the soil they inhabit in ways that sustain their existence in that very habitat. Simply put, the worms construct an environmental niche that increases their chances of survival. In philosophy of mind, the idea of niche construction has been applied similarly to designate the various processes whereby humans manipulate the material, social, cultural, and epistemic environment to support and enhance their psychological and experiential capabilities (see Clark, 2006; Colombetti & Krueger, 2015; Sterelny, 2010; Sutton, Harris, Keil, & Barnier, 2010). Like the situated approach to mind, niche construction emphasizes our own activeness – both individually and collectively – in influencing how we come to think and feel.

Basically, the aforementioned insights boil down to the claim that *we build niches to scaffold our minds*. To gain more insight into how this happens, we may distinguish between niches based on their primary *domains of influence* – that is, in terms of the particular capacities and experiences that they scaffold (Krueger, 2014a; Maiese, 2016; Sutton, 2016; Saarinen, 2019; Saarinen, forthcoming). *Cognitive* niche construction consists in developing and using environmental resources to support and enhance problem solving, reasoning, decision making, remembering, and other such mental activities. Think, for instance, of satellite navigation systems that enable us to find the optimal route from one place to another and the calculators that help us compute the journey's expenses. Nowadays, of course, smartphones scaffold our cognitive capacities more extensively than any other material resources routinely available. *Affective* niche construction, in turn, takes place when the environment is manipulated to scaffold emotions, moods, atmospheric feelings, and other states and processes belonging to the 'affective realm' (see Chapter 1). We listen to music to get into the groove, engage in therapy to manage our anxieties, and participate in sports to feel the thrill of competition. Obviously, the niches we inhabit and the environmental resources they consist of need not operate on a simple either/or basis. Indeed, they often scaffold cognition and affect *simultaneously*, albeit in different ways and to varying extents. Nor do we need to delimit the effects of scaffolds to just cognition and affect; niches also enable and support different kinds of *actions* and *behaviors*. Even so, the suggested distinction between the two domains is conceptually useful, as it enables us to analyze in closer detail the cognitive/affective aspects of scaffolding, and to identify which of the two, if either, is the primary target of influence in any given niche.

At this point it is worth noting that, in contrast to the cognitive domain, 'affective niche construction' and 'affective scaffolding' are relatively novel theoretical developments, having first been introduced systematically into philosophy of mind as recently as 2015 by Giovanna Colombetti and Joel Krueger in their article "Scaffoldings of the affective mind". In their account, scaffolding depends on two key factors, namely the *active manipulation* of environmental elements and the *mutual influence* between the agent and the environment. To put this in slightly different terms, Colombetti and Krueger accentuate (a) the extent to which affective experience involves "actively modifying one's environment for the sake of one's affective life itself", and (b) how this amounts to "affective niches" which, in essence, establish "organism-environment couplings (mutual influences) that enable the realization of specific affective states" (2015, p. 1160). In sum, then, Colombetti and Krueger maintain that grasping the experiential structure of moods, emotions, etc. requires an analysis of "the ways in which agents engineer their affective environments – that is, create affective niches – and in so doing let these environments influence their affective states in an ongoing way" (p. 1160).

Because 'affective scaffolding' is still in its early stages of theoretical development, its conceptual boundaries are somewhat unsettled. For instance, no cogent arguments have been made for criteria that clearly distinguish scaffolded affects from non-scaffolded ones; nor, for that matter, has any agreement been reached on whether such clear-cut criteria are even desirable or necessary (for discussion, see Krueger, 2018; Saarinen, forthcoming; Slaby, 2016; Sutton, 2016). I will not dive deeper into the technicalities of this philosophical issue here. For the purposes of this study, I simply adopt a broad and pragmatic position on scaffolding – a position that should not be expected to distinguish between scaffolded and non-scaffolded states. Instead, the concept is used to identify and elaborate on what is considered to be a relatively *perpetual* feature of affective experience. In this view, the world we inhabit is a multiform niche with which we (must) constantly interact – in one way or another and with varying degrees of personal deliberation, self-awareness, and control – to influence our affective experience. Thus, more often than not, we find ourselves in niches that scaffold the way we feel.

I take my lead in this respect from John Sutton, who has challenged the notion of a bare, *essentially non-scaffolded* mind:

> For the sciences of the mind there is no reason to think that the essential level of analysis should be the performance of the naked brain or the unscaffolded mind. Rather, human psychology is most characteristically seen and experienced in our tangled, dynamic interrelations with social, environmental, and technological systems. Instead of stripping away the scaffolding and the multiple influences in search of something pristine beneath, *the explanatory task is to document and trace the many forms of scaffolding* and the shifting cognitive constructions they support.
>
> (Sutton, 2016, p. 197, my italics)

Moreover, referring specifically to affect, Sutton notes how "our moods and emotions are constantly shaped, given precision or flavor, by way of social uptake, culturally-specific caring practices, or self-induced rituals and habits such as listening to music, going to a particular place, or just having another coffee" (2016, p. 192). This is a broader and less restrictive position on scaffolding than maintaining that we *sometimes* interact with the environment with the *express intention* of modifying our psychological and experiential lives. It instead entails that the mind is always already intertwined with, and supported by, a complex and multiform network of scaffoldings.

Sutton's view highlights how ubiquitous affective scaffolding is in our everyday lives. That being so, the best way to apply the concept is to systematically 'trace' and 'document' how experience is scaffolded in the various practical contexts and situations in which it unfolds. In this way, a rigorous and comprehensive analysis of affective scaffolding can provide significant insight into the ways in which any given affective state is environmentally enabled and supported. In the next section, I will argue that a *multidimensional* model of the scaffolded mind works particularly well for this purpose (see Sterelny, 2010; Colombetti & Krueger, 2015; Saarinen, forthcoming).

However, before introducing the multidimensional model and applying it to painting, a brief theoretical qualification is in order. The promotion of affective scaffolding as a significant and pervasive phenomenon is strongly motivated by so-called externalist views of the mind. To explain affectivity, externalism aims to substitute theories that focus on internal and typically brain-centric organismic mechanisms with accounts that emphasize integrated organism–environment couplings and interactions (Colombetti & Krueger, 2015). Within this externalist framework, several scholars have advanced the thesis of *extended affectivity*, which holds that environmental elements/resources can become *ontologically constitutive* parts of affective states, in addition to merely enabling, supporting, and modifying them (for further discussion, see Colombetti, 2017a; Colombetti & Roberts, 2015; Krueger, 2014b; Krueger & Szanto, 2016; Maiese, 2016; Slaby, 2014; Stephan et al., 2014; Sterelny, 2010). The proponent of affective scaffolding can, however, remain neutral about this contested issue, as the key premises of 'scaffolding' hold regardless of whether or not extension occurs in the suggested sense. I will adopt this moderate position here and leave the thornier ontological debate aside.

Painting and multidimensional affective scaffolding

As suggested, we can add significant detail to how the scaffolded mind works by investigating it along several interrelated *dimensions*. I will discuss scaffolded affectivity specifically in terms of *elemental structure*, *temporality*, *reciprocality*, *individuality/collectivity*, *trust*, *individualization/entrenchment*, and *intent*. While this multidimensional model does not necessarily exhaust all aspects of scaffolding, it does enable us to examine with clarity and precision how affective experience depends on and varies according to certain environmental circumstances and interactions, and how particular environmental resources can be actively used to bring about certain affective effects. As such, it also helps us to understand how painting and paintings can function as significant affective scaffolds to artists, enabling them to feel – in a unique manner – things that would otherwise be difficult, if not indeed impossible, for them to feel.

Elemental structure

Let us focus first on the structural elements of affective niches. These elements are, quite simply, all the *environmental resources* that can be manipulated and used for scaffolding purposes. A broad distinction can be made, for instance, between *material* and *social* resources (Krueger, 2018; Sutton, 2016). Material resources encompass the inanimate world of things, including natural objects and man-made artefacts, tools, and instruments, and both natural and manufactured places and spaces, such as wildlife sanctuaries, public buildings, and private living rooms. Social resources, in turn, consist in the people we interact with, be they individuals, groups, or larger collectives. Again, the suggested division is somewhat simplistic, considering how often niches are not only composed of *both* types of resources but also of *other* types that do not fit neatly under either, such as shared cultural symbols. The takeaway point is that, as long as they enable and regulate our affective states, scaffolds can be anything from psychotropic pills to workplace environments and sociocultural norms (see Colombetti & Krueger, 2015; Slaby, 2016).

The diversity of possible resources means that affective scaffolds vary widely in regard to their specificity, materiality, perceivability, and manipulability. I have elsewhere introduced the term *concreteness* to refer to the extent to which a given resource is distinguishable and intelligible as something with which one can tangibly interact (Saarinen, 2019). To get a better idea of what this means, let us first consider an instance of *non*-concrete scaffolding: the act of taking a vacation to cheer oneself up (an example of affective scaffolding given by Colombetti & Krueger, 2015, p. 1162). As I see it, vacations are best understood as sequences of events that unfold over relatively extended periods of time and involve countless interactions with various resources in numerous different settings. That being so, it is rather difficult to grasp the overall structure of the 'vacation niche', and indeed to discern which scaffoldings are particularly relevant to cheering oneself up. There does not seem to be any distinct type of agent–environment coupling or mutual influence operative in this case. In contrast, consider petting a dog to relax and to soothe oneself (and the dog); here we find an active engagement with a physically distinct and clearly specifiable object, and, moreover, an agent–resource interaction to which the positive feeling can clearly be attributed. As such, it is a prime example of concrete affective scaffolding.

Turning to the elemental structure of painterly niches, it is self-evident that paintings are – at least in the common, traditional view – relatively clearly demarcated material things (for a more unorthodox view, see, e.g., Graw, 2018). They are objects made of paints and other substances that have been applied to solid surfaces. Hence the affective scaffolding provided by paintings is straightforwardly concrete in the previously specified sense. To add more substance to this observation, we could analyze how paintings scaffold feeling in virtue of their *distinctive* material features, and, moreover, examine whether these characteristic features of paintings support particular kinds of affective states. We might, for instance, consider the size of the canvas; the visual, olfactory, and tactile qualities of paint itself (see Chapter 4); or the ways in which certain colors and compositions scaffold specific feelings. As regards size, the way the body is involved in painting a large canvas versus a small one is presumably quite different, which may in turn affect the degree and nature of feelings of merging with and inhabiting the space of the painting.

In sum, paintings are self-evidently concrete material resources. When perceived from an objective, third-person point of view, not only are they *clearly demarcated* objects but also *inanimate* ones. However, the situation can look surprisingly different when we also consider paintings from the first-person experiential perspective of painters themselves. From this subjective viewpoint, the boundaries and lifelessness of paintings are no longer such clear-cut issues. During the creative process, many artists relate to their paintings not just as material objects but also, in a very special sense, as autonomous agents or living others. In this fashion, besides being material resources, paintings can simultaneously be experienced by their makers as *social* or *interpersonal* resources as well. Moreover, the boundaries between one's self and one's painting can be felt to dissolve, leading to more or less intense experiences of fusion with the work. I will discuss these peculiar phenomena further in Chapters 4 and 5, respectively.

Temporality

In addition to incorporating numerous possible environmental elements, affective niches can operate on *various timescales* (Colombetti & Krueger, 2015; Griffiths & Scarantino, 2009; Sutton, 2016). When scaffolding is *synchronic*, the relevant resource is 'set up' and put to use at a particular point in time to support concurrent affective experience. A simple example of this would be engaging in intimate conversation with a friend to sort out one's ongoing difficult feelings. Other scaffoldings operate *diachronically* over longer periods of time. Colombetti and Krueger note, for instance, how religious and spiritual spaces are typically "designed to induce a variety of feelings, such as faith, hope, awe, love, compassion, and guilt, with the aid of disparate material objects and practices" (2015, p. 1171–1172). Such niches are often built and developed to operate intergenerationally, and indeed over time tend to "lead to culturally and socially different affective experiences and modalities of conduct" (p. 1172). Overall, the functioning of longer-term niches can be analyzed on various timelines (see Sutton, 2016). *Phylogenetic* analysis traces how niche construction figures in the evolutionary development and diversification of the human species, whereas *ontogenic* analysis focuses on individual persons' developmental trajectories. *Cultural-historical* analysis in turn seeks to disclose the ways in which niches are culturally created, sustained, and transmitted from one generation to the next via norms, institutions, accumulated expertise, traditions, rituals, and so on.

The temporal course of painting can also be delineated in various ways. Besides the actual application of paint to canvas, painting may involve, among other things, buying and preparing the necessary materials, gathering ideas and inspiration from different sources, and mulling over the work outside the studio. Whichever way we choose to frame the process of painting, it is necessarily an activity that is *diachronically* scaffolded. To give an example, the painting traditions with which the artist engages, either critically or approvingly, consciously or unconsciously, and the kinds of artistic self-understandings that these traditions encourage or discourage will necessarily affect the artist's experience of painting. Just think of the difference between exploring subjective emotional states via Romantic/Expressionist painting versus the impersonal and predetermined Minimalist approach of, say, Frank Stella in his *Black Paintings* series (see Chapter 6). Simply put, painters do not paint in a vacuum. They are embedded in art historical and cultural contexts that enable, sustain, and make intelligible certain kinds of affective relations to their paintings.

Without diminishing the significance of diachronic scaffolding in painting, in the following chapters I discuss the artist's affective experience primarily with respect to *synchronic* engagement with paintings: the process of making marks on the canvas, appraising those marks, making more marks in response, and so on. I will focus on how this ongoing material interaction between the painter and the painting scaffolds concurrent affective experience. Yet another way of putting this is that I will mainly analyze the real-time relational aspects of affective scaffolding rather than the longer-term and more broadly cultural and historical scaffoldings that operate in the background, as it were. With that said, I will enquire into how various *ontogenetic* factors contribute to synchronic affective scaffolding in painting. Moreover, I will have something to say about how painting can, in the longer run, transform and organize one's affectively based way of relating to the world as a whole (see Chapter 7). In this sense, my analysis brings a considerable element of individually focused historical understanding to the matter.

Reciprocality

The previously discussed dimensions of structure and temporality provide a general descriptive framework for the functioning of affective niches. They constitute the basic environmental and temporal parameters within which scaffolding operates. By homing in on the rich variety of actual *agent–resource interactions*, we can identify further dimensions that are key to scaffolding situations. One such variable is the degree to which any given case of scaffolding involves *causal reciprocality* or *mutual influence* between the agent and the relevant environmental resource (Colombetti & Krueger, 2015; Krueger, 2018; Heersmink & Sutton, 2018). Sometimes resources operate more or less unidirectionally to scaffold experience, like when one chooses a soft item of clothing to feel safe and cozy (example from Colombetti & Krueger, 2015, p. 1163). The way the clothing makes the agent feel does not bring about any change in the piece of clothing itself. In other cases, the relevant resource is much more 'responsive' to the agent's actions. For example, when an improvising musician plays music that affects her current feeling, that feeling will influence what she improvises next, and so on in cyclical fashion (Krueger & Szanto, 2016, p. 867). Here the resource – the music being produced – plays a reciprocal role in the ongoing scaffolding activity. With an eye on these kinds of differences, I have introduced the term *robustness* to refer to the extent to which a given instance of affective scaffolding manifests synchronous causal bidirectionality between the agent and the affective resource (Saarinen, 2019).

In this respect, it is striking how many artists and art researchers have portrayed painting as a two-way dialogical interaction between the painter and the progressing work of art (see, e.g., Ehrenzweig, 1967; Elkins, 2000; Hagman, 2005; Milner, 1957; Nelson & Rawlings, 2007; Newton, 2008; Rose, 1980; Townsend, 2019; Wentworth, 2005; Wright, 2009). This notion is especially widely held by those who regard painting as an open-ended process of exploration rather than the execution of predetermined ideas or intentions. When the artist does not possess fixed and precise knowledge of how the work will turn out, she must remain attentive and responsive to its emerging, cue-like features. Under such circumstances, the painting is more likely to be experienced as an interlocutor: a presence that responds to the artist's painterly gestures by shutting down certain possibilities while opening up others, and by resisting, suggesting, or even demanding further courses of action.

Depictions of painting as a dialogue support the notion that it is a synchronous, causally bidirectional process. The artist actively manipulates a material object so that it induces readjustments in her prior intentions towards that object, which in turn prompts her to respond with further modifying actions, and so on cyclically until the work is considered complete. Importantly, many of the affects invoked by the creative process depend completely on how this give-and-take pans out. One such feeling is that of getting the painting to work or to resonate (see Chapter 6). Suffice it to say at this point that feelings of this kind qualify as *robustly* scaffolded affects by virtue of being enabled and supported by the highly bidirectional activity of painting. In slightly different terms, the developing painting becomes part of an integrated painter–painting feedback loop that structures the artist's ongoing emotional experience. Some affects scaffolded in this manner (for example, elevated mood) may in turn guide the creative process by signaling whether it is progressing in a satisfactory direction (see Anderson & Hausman, 1992; Collingwood, 1958; Ehrenzweig, 1967; Nelson & Rawlings, 2007).

Individuality/collectivity

Besides reciprocality, scaffolding situations vary along the dimension of *individuality-collectivity* (Colombetti & Krueger, 2015; Sterelny, 2010). On one end of this spectrum we find individuals interacting with singular environmental resources to scaffold their own feelings, such as devising a personal playlist on a music streaming platform to evoke and sustain a specific mood. On the other end of the spectrum we find situations where agents act together within collectively structured niches to produce shared affective effects. For example, fans at sporting events participate in chants, songs, and choreographies that are not only meant to intimidate the opposition but also to produce feelings of group cohesion, strength, and an overall 'buzz' for everyone involved.

As I pointed out with respect to temporal diachronicity, painting is embedded in a certain historical and cultural context. In this sense, the activity of painting necessarily takes place in a collectively structured niche, indirectly as this may be. Painting can also be organized collectively in a more direct, here-and-now fashion. Consider Damien Hirst's famous 'spot paintings', which were produced through a process of distributed responsibility. Hirst himself took the role of organizer-overseer while a crew of aides actually painted most of the works. (As a critical riposte, David Hockney advertised his own contemporaneous exhibition with the announcement: "All the works here were made by the artist himself, personally".) Whatever one makes of this, assistants/apprentices have contributed in various ways and to various extents to artworks from Michelangelo and Rembrandt to Andy Warhol and Jeff Koons. There are also artists who work together on the same paintings *simultaneously*, for example, the painter twins Marina and Irina Fabrizius (www.fabrizius2.de). Arguably, these various collective ways of making art each enable and sustain different kinds of affective atmospheres, shared emotions, and individual feelings.

For the sake of clarity and incisiveness, in this study I will concentrate solely on individual painters working on their own paintings. This practical limitation marks paintings off from affective resources that are being created jointly or by others. A personal, one-to-one relation to artwork will presumably support very different kinds of feelings than more collective ways of working. My choice thus allows me to focus on affects that are scaffolded specifically by reciprocal interactions between the individual painter and the developing work.

Trust

It is also important to note that there are varying levels of *trust* involved in scaffolding interactions (Colombetti & Krueger, 2015; Sterelny, 2010). Here, trust refers to the perceived *reliability* of a given environmental resource in supporting particular experiences or bringing about certain affective effects. Put otherwise, scaffolds can be deemed trustworthy if they influence one's affective states in experientially proven and fairly predictable ways. For instance, some people feel that participating in shared religious practices is a reliable way of bolstering their sense of security, purpose, and belonging. Sometimes strong dependence on a certain resource may develop into outright *addiction* (Colombetti & Krueger, 2015, p. 1162). When their careers end, professional athletes may find it extremely difficult to live without the adrenaline kick of rigorous competition and the camaraderie of locker room culture. They are, quite simply, left with an emotional void that desperately needs filling in one way or another. In sum, repeated interactions with dependable resources often develop into habits – or in more extreme cases, into addictions – that range from the beneficial to the downright detrimental.

Painters also come to expect and value certain affects during the creative process. These may include, for instance, feelings of absorption, emancipation, surprise, harmonious attunement, omnipotence, and vitality. Through the accumulation of painterly experience, artists come to trust that the creative dialogue will eventually give rise to such desired feelings. Indeed, painters are drawn to their work largely because they perceive their developing paintings as sufficiently *dependable* resources for special affective states. This does not, however, mean that reaching these states is effortless or automatic. For example, the feeling of getting the painting to work typically requires persistent effort and lengthy processes of trial and error (see Chapter 6). The painter must trust in her own ability to find the right solutions when faced with unavoidable creative blocks and frustrating setbacks.

As mentioned, in the case of addiction, the individual comes to perceive a specific resource as an irreplaceable scaffold for highly valued feelings and is thus compelled to return to it repeatedly. I believe this applies to many artists' nearly compulsive need to paint. In fact, as George Hagman (2005, p. 72) has pointed out, painters do not become addicted to any *single* feeling so much as to the *entire creative cycle*. It is the affectively multifaceted and often laborious process of seeking, achieving, losing, and regaining that 'special something' in painting that proves to be so compelling. Moreover, once the creative effort is completed successfully, the artist may experience herself as renewed and revitalized (Hagman, 2005, p. 68). That this is such a hard-fought victory only adds to the intensity of these feelings. In this manner, the painterly endeavor can become addictively rewarding.

Individualization and entrenchment

There is also variation in the *individualization* of environmental resources – that is, in the extent to which they are adapted and fitted by agents to suit their personal purposes, preferences, and habitual activities (Colombetti &

Krueger, 2015; Sterelny, 2010). On a material level, this is illustrated by the relationships that professionals and skilled experts develop with the tools and instruments of their specific crafts or trades – for example, when carpenters customize their tool belts to suit their personal needs, habits, and working methods. Sometimes replacing such highly individualized resources with similar yet non-individualized ones will considerably alter the agent's scaffolded capacities and experiences, as the new resources just don't seem to feel right or work in the same fluid manner.

Many painters also customize their artistic resources to suit their personal preferences and needs. This applies not only to the brushes, knives, sponges, and other tools that are used in painting but also to the broader environmental niche in which the creative cycle is realized. The latter is, in effect, the artist's *studio* or *atelier*. The personal selection and adjustment of lighting, material props, visual prompts, auditory aids, etc. thus creates a space that enables and protects creativity – and its concomitant affects – in a highly individualized way.

Individualized resources can also become experienced as *deeply ingrained* or *entrenched* parts of oneself and what one does. Consider, again, the professional musician and her instrument. Over time, the musician may develop an individualized feel for a particular instrument, which in turn enables her to play it with great finesse. In addition to this, and perhaps more significantly, playing music can become so deeply ingrained into the musician's affective-expressive repertoire that losing access to the instrument or the ability to play it amounts to an incapability to feel certain moods and emotions altogether (Colombetti & Krueger, 2015, p. 1164). Thus, not only are certain tools or instruments ingrained into the creative self; the overall activity of creating with certain materials and in specific ways may also become entrenched into one's basic sense of being.

In the same way, the activity of painting can become irreplaceably integrated into the painter's overall affective landscape. For many painters, painting may well be the sole means of experiencing certain desirable and valued feelings. In short, artistic creativity scaffolds feelings that would otherwise be difficult, if not impossible, to attain. This notion is supported, for example, by painter Maisa Kela's description of the experiential possibilities that painting discloses. She writes:

> Painting can alleviate anxiety. It's soothing because you converse with yourself, you don't need another person. You can grasp something

> about yourself that is not possible otherwise. Instead of talking with a therapist, you converse with a picture. The painting process is a mirror that helps you relax and gives you new insight about yourself.
>
> (Huttula, 2017, p. 163; my translation)

Intent

Finally, it should be noted that supporting and regulating affect via scaffolding does not necessarily require *conscious intent* on the scaffolded individual's part (Colombetti & Krueger, 2015; Slaby, 2016). To a large extent, we go through our everyday lives habitually and unreflectively, and this applies to numerous scaffolding interactions as well. One may, for example, quite unreflectively execute a series of customary morning routines – turn on certain lights, have a fixed amount of coffee, read the paper's sections in a specific order – just to get the day going on the right affective note. Furthermore, our affects are often scaffolded via others' actions and outside forces, too, even if we are not fully aware of this or do not consent to it (Krueger, forthcoming; Slaby, 2016). We only need to consider how deeply and extensively mobile technology – as the 'technology that goes where the user goes' – has pervaded our experiential lives. This may, as a negative consequence, compel us to feel constantly and overbearingly connected to our working-life duties and commitments (Slaby, 2016, p. 10). Thus, whether or not we are aware of it, environmental niches continuously influence the way we think and feel.

This also means that when painters set out to paint, they need not be *explicitly aware* of hoping to achieve certain feelings through their creative activities. During the course of painting, their thoughts and attention will most likely be on the artwork itself and on the practical challenges that it poses. Nevertheless, when artists *do* contemplate their praxis from a more detached standpoint, they commonly recognize certain recurrent affects as pleasurable, valuable, and hence *desirable*. For instance, the feelings of flow and getting the painting to work are frequently identified as high points of painterly experience, and as vitalizing feelings that make the whole effort worthwhile. Achieving such states is one of the main reasons that painters begin to labor over their paintings in the first place. In sum, painters clearly prize certain feelings in painterly engagement and seek their realization, even if they largely do so habitually and unconsciously.

Concluding remarks

In this chapter, I have suggested that painting is not only about producing finished artworks, about expressing or giving form to experience, or about communicating certain contents. It is equally about the creation of a niche in which certain desirable and otherwise elusive feelings are enabled, realized, and valued. To support this claim, I have examined affective scaffolding – both in general and in relation to painting – in terms of elemental structure, temporality, reciprocality, individuality/collectivity, trust, individualization/entrenchment, and intent. The aim of this discussion has been twofold: first, to demonstrate that the scaffolded mind is a multidimensional phenomenon and that scaffolding interactions accordingly come in a wide variety of forms, and second, to clarify and delimit the scope of my upcoming analyses of specific painterly affects (in Chapters 4–6). In discussing painting, I have placed particular emphasis on the dimensional features of concreteness, synchronicity, robustness, individuality, and dependability. In this view, affective scaffolding in painting is constituted by *synchronic reciprocality* between an *active individual agent* and a resource that is *sufficiently distinct* and *reliably efficacious* with regard to the agent's desired affect.

With this specification in mind, I want to conclude with a few thoughts on what sets painting apart from other forms of affective scaffolding. Joel Krueger and Thomas Szanto have pointed out that different affective resources "have different properties, formats, and functions, and thus invite different forms of engagement, integration, and emotional enhancement" (2016, p. 865). Paintings can accordingly be investigated as resources that enable special affective experiences and forms of engagement due to their characteristic properties and functions. So, what precisely makes them special? Three features deserve separate mention. First, during painting, paintings differ from most affective resources in that they are in the *process of being created by the agent whose affects they scaffold*. This sets them apart from resources that are already existing and available for scaffolding. The latter encompass all 'ready-made' resources that do not need to be specially created or devised by the individual for scaffolding purposes.

Second, not only are paintings in the process of being created, but, in the suggested dialogical framework, are being created specifically by means of *open-ended interaction*. This is because painting usually aims to achieve or bring about something that is not fully known or foreseen at the outset. This distinguishes paintings from resources that are likewise being created by individual agents but involve chiefly predetermined notions of expected outcomes and more fixed procedures for achieving them (e.g., making pizza to lower one's level of tension, as per Colombetti, 2017b).

At this point, one might point out that other forms of artistic activity – such as composing music, writing poetry, and sculpting – also scaffold the artist's affect via open-ended, one-on-one interaction with resources that are simultaneously being created. This is true. However, what sets these different creative forms of scaffolding apart from each other and also influences the quality and types of affects they scaffold is their *characteristic materiality*. In a very basic sense, it *feels* different to work with sounds, written words, clay, paint, and so on. Each medium has its unique sensory-perceptual properties and possibilities for manipulation, and thus invites different forms of engagement, integration, and emotional enhancement. For example, some painters describe their canvases as skin-like (see Chapter 4). Surely this kind of material engagement engenders very different kinds of feelings of the aliveness of artworks than, say, playing and hearing music.

To be absolutely clear, I do not mean to imply that the robust, dependable, concrete, and individually accentuated scaffolding that I have specified for this study is the only kind of scaffolding that warrants recognition. Instead, I have delineated the given, relatively restricted form of affective scaffolding for purposes of analytical focus and cogency. Returning to the issue of conceptual usefulness, I believe that within these parameters, the concept of scaffolding discloses something new and significant about the ways in which affective experience is supported by painting. It also enables us to expand on this revelation in a rigorous, comprehensive, and illuminating way. Needless to say, my approach also has its limitations. I readily admit that it leaves out various aspects of what painting is and can be. Given that painters paint for different reasons and in different ways, I do not want to give the impression that all painting necessarily amounts to affective scaffolding in the specified sense. For the same reason, I also want to avoid making any universal or normative claims about the essence of artistic creativity. Having said that, I do believe that many painters relate to their works and experience the creative process in ways I have discussed earlier. In sum, my more moderate premise is that *under certain conditions*, painting *can* function as a significant affective scaffold to painters.

All in all, the theories of niche construction and scaffolding provide useful tools for analyzing the *formal* aspects of agent–environment situatedness and interaction. Within the multidimensional framework we can, as Sutton urges, trace and document the many forms of scaffolding that support our affective lives, painting included. However, what is missing from this formal approach is a proper understanding of what drives the multitude of scaffolding interactions or, more specifically, of how these scaffoldings are organized by earlier object relations and motivated by unconscious needs and concerns. To fill in this gap, I will next turn to psychoanalysis. Drawing from its rich theoretical tradition, I will analyze why painters seek certain feelings through painting. I will also elaborate on the unique, interpersonal way in which paintings come to scaffold these feelings.

Chapter 3

The developmental roots of creative being and painting

In the previous chapter, I used the concepts of niche construction and affective scaffolding to argue that painters paint in order to influence the way they feel. Viewed in this light, painting involves setting up a niche in which paintings-in-progress scaffold the artist's ongoing emotions, moods, and other affective states. I also presented the multidimensional framework of scaffolding to illuminate several noteworthy aspects of the affectively charged painter–painting relationship. However, these theoretical approaches can only take us so far in grasping the nature of painterly affectivity. For one thing, they do not tell us why certain affective states become important and desirable in painting. Vice versa, they do not explain how the activity of painting develops into a crucial resource for such feelings. Hence, we need a complementary account of why painters value and seek certain feelings in relation to their artwork, and how paintings in turn come to function as scaffolds for such feelings.

I address these issues in this chapter by examining the developmental background of painting. My basic premise is that early ontogenesis shapes later creative activity in various significant ways. From this point of view, painting can be seen as a creative form of object-relating that is deeply rooted in the earliest interactions between the infant and the caretaking environment. This also means that painters come to their here-and-now interactions with paintings from a lengthy and complexly patterned background of personal affective scaffoldings. In short, individual developmental history influences what painters seek to feel via painting, and how they come to achieve this.

I will elaborate on this idea as follows. I first discuss how individuals are born into caretaking niches which, from the start, provide developmentally crucial affective scaffoldings. More specifically, I examine how early infant–caregiver interactions instill in the baby the basic capacity and confidence to *engage creatively* with the world. From this starting point, the creative attitude gradually extends and diversifies to encompass a variety of external objects, including works of art. Moreover, at this early stage, several *core concerns* pertaining to one's being are set into motion – concerns which inevitably, yet mostly unconsciously, continue to bear upon adult experience and behavior. I introduce four such concerns, namely, how to relate *subjective* and *objective* realities; how to demarcate between *me* and *not-me*; how to cope with *separation* and the associated need for meaningful *connection* with others; and how to achieve and strengthen the sense of being *fully alive*. Overall, I argue that painting enables the artist to attend to and play with these interrelated concerns creatively. I also suggest that many of the feelings most valued in the painting process are inextricably linked to how this existential play pans out.

Forging a creative world-relation

In its original form, niche construction theory examines the ways in which organisms modify their surroundings to influence their own, their species', and other species' fitness. It illuminates how active environmental manipulation affects the survival and reproduction rate of competing types in a population, and thus seeks to explain, on an evolutionary timescale, *selective* genetic variation. To complement this view, Karola Stotz (2010, 2017) has promoted the concept of *developmental* niche construction. It aims to clarify, on an ontogenetic timescale, both the maturation of species-typical traits and the production of novel within-species variation. This approach to niche construction foregrounds the non-genetic inheritance and modification of resources that support life-cyclical development. According to Stotz, human developmental niche construction has become especially complex and resource-demanding due to our species' increased brain size and lengthy postnatal immaturity. It requires intensive parental care, nurture, playing, social learning, and so on. The ramifications of these early processes are diverse and far-reaching. As Stotz puts it, the developmental niche has powerful effects on the type of nature one develops with regard to mental health, sociality, and morality. I adopt this basic idea and suggest that we add both creativity and affectivity to the aforementioned key areas of developmental influence.

Within the developmental niche, the infant–caregiver dyad is an outstanding topic of interest. Colombetti and Krueger also discuss its role in establishing the capacity for (later) interpersonal affective scaffoldings (2015, pp. 1167–1169). They suggest that, initially, the key affective function of the dyad is to enable, support, and regulate feelings that the infant cannot occasion and sustain on his own, especially positive feelings like being soothed and satisfied. Simply put, the caregiver attunes to the infant's occurrent state and responds accordingly to scaffold his ongoing affective experience (see also Taipale, 2016). In this scenario, the baby is not just a passive recipient of one-way affective modulation. Rather, as Colombetti and Krueger are quick to point out, the infant plays an active role in dyadic interaction, and can therefore be seen "to participate in the construction of a specific infant-caregiver affective niche" (2015, p. 1168).

The formation of *trust* is paramount in early dyadic interaction, and also exemplifies its bidirectional nature fittingly. Based on findings in empirical research, Colombetti and Krueger suggest that infants begin to differentiate between reliable and unreliable sources of affective feedback from very early on (2015, pp. 1168–1169). In favorable circumstances, the infant's primary caregivers come to serve as familiar and trustworthy scaffolds. Thus, the baby learns to actively seek them out for affective support and regulation. In more adverse conditions, however, the baby might not attain much confidence in the scaffolding ability of its caregivers, nor of others more generally. In the case of severe maternal depression, for instance, infants come to distrust not only their mothers' faces but also the faces of others, and their capacity to decipher affective facial expressions is accordingly diminished (Colombetti & Krueger, 2015, p. 1679; see also Varga & Krueger, 2013). Infants affected in this way are likely to abandon the unreliable resources and search elsewhere for much-needed affective feedback.

A basic sense of trust in other persons and their availability for scaffolding purposes is thus laid down in the early developmental niche. But this does not yet cover the range of primary trust. At this stage, a more general sense of being able to depend on objects for psychological sustenance and enrichment is also established. Put broadly, this sense concerns one's capacity to modify the environment at large in personally meaningful ways. In psychological health, the external world need not be submissively complied with, but is rather experienced as something that can be remolded to accommodate one's desires, concerns, fantasies, and the like, and, through this, to reflect them back in personally significant form. That is to say, sensitively attuned dyadic interaction instills in the infant the confidence that the world can be *engaged with creatively*. A psychologically barren and unresponsive developmental niche will accordingly undermine the development of this confidence to varying degrees. I will now shift theoretical gears and elaborate on this matter from a psychoanalytical point of view.

We are born with a tendency to explore and interact with our surroundings. The evolution of this predisposition into a full-blown creative world-relation is not, however, a foregone conclusion. It is a developmental achievement that presupposes sufficient nurture in the early caretaking niche, and, once established, may also be disrupted or lost. This, in a nutshell, was the main insight of Donald W. Winnicott, the pediatrician and psychoanalyst who authored one of the most evocative accounts of creativity to date, and whose ideas I will build upon here. Winnicott's pivotal claim was that creativity is based on and unfolds in an *intermediate area of experience* between subjective psychic life and objective shared reality. In developing this idea, he introduced several novel concepts, most notably those of 'transitional object', 'transitional phenomena', and 'potential space', but also refashioned more familiar ones, including 'illusion', 'mirroring', and 'playing', to better suit his purposes. On the whole, Winnicott combined these concepts into a highly original and occasionally enigmatic account of creativity and creative living.

It is worth noting three general features of Winnicott's conception of creativity before delving deeper into its specifics. First, he discusses creativity mostly as a way of *experientially relating* to the external world at large (1971, pp. 65–85). The type of creativity that Winnicott has in mind is thus not limited to artistic work or to other self-evidently creative activities, nor is it to be identified solely with respect to observable creative products or achievements. It is, in short, a way of *being* or *existing*. Second, instead of focusing on the instinctual or intrapsychic elements of creativity, as per more traditional psychoanalytic approaches, Winnicott highlights the necessity of sufficient *environmental provision*, both in quality and frequency, in forging a creative world-relation. As he puts it,

> at this point where creativity either comes into being or does not come into being (or alternatively is lost) the theoretician must take the environment into account, and *no statement that concerns the individual as an isolate* can touch this central problem of the source of creativity. (p. 71, my italics)

In this respect, Winnicott's conceptualization parallels the notion of the situated mind, which grasps mental activity as fundamentally codetermined by the environmental context in which it occurs (see Chapter 2). His approach therefore lends itself nicely to the conceptual framework of niche construction and affective scaffolding.

Finally, Winnicott discusses the origins of creativity mainly in terms of infant–*mother* interaction. In his view, for the baby, the mother is the first environment – both biologically and psychologically. This maternal emphasis might strike present-day readers as overly colored and even tainted by conservative and outdated views on family, gender, and gender roles. In order to engage with Winnicott's thinking and to discern which aspects of his theory are still applicable today, one may indeed need to overcome several gender-related terminological and theoretical obstacles. On the other hand, as Jan Abram encapsulates it, for Winnicott "the concept of mother as environment" also includes "the father, siblings, the extended family, society, and the world at large" (2007, p. 217). Even so, in explicit recognition of the multiform nature of the caretaking niche, I will mainly use the more inclusive terms 'caregiver' and 'caretaking environment' when discussing early interaction, and by eschewing gendered expressions will try to avoid any possible misconceptions. Only when quoting Winnicott or Winnicottian theorists directly, or when the mother has been specified for good reason, will I use 'maternal' terms.

So, then, what is Winnicott's take on the etiology of creative being? As indicated, he locates the developmental roots of creativity in the earliest contacts between the caretaking environment and the infant. He observes how environmental provision involves, at first, near complete and exact adaptation to the infant's needs. Such attentive attunement evokes in the infant the *illusion* of magical control over the mother's breast – which, besides being an actual part of the mother's body, encompasses the overall "technique of mothering", including possible bottle-feeding (Winnicott, 1971, pp. 10–12). Subjectively, the baby feels he "creates" the breast as it emerges to satisfy his hunger right when he needs it to. Winnicott describes this sequence as follows:

> [A]n infant is . . . capable of conceiving of the idea of something that would meet the growing need that arises out of instinctual tension. The infant cannot be said to know at first what is to be created. At this point in time the mother presents herself. . . . The mother's adaptation

> to the infant's needs, when good enough, gives the infant the *illusion* that there is an external reality that corresponds to the infant's own capacity to create. In other words, there is an overlap between what the mother supplies and what the child might conceive of. To the observer, the child perceives what the mother actually presents, but this is not the whole truth. The infant perceives the breast only in so far as a breast could be created just there and then.
>
> (Winnicott, 1971, p. 12)

Winnicott calls this early dyadic actualization of the infant's creative impulse *primary creativity* (1971, pp. 10–12). He also suggests that this type of creativity unfolds in a state of merger with the caregiving (part-) object, namely, the mother or the mother's breast (pp. 14, 47–48, 96–97, 107). It is beside the point to speculate whether or not the baby's earliest experience is categorically one of absolute fusion with its caregiver(s) or the world in general. We may just presume that experience at this stage is regularly accentuated by feelings of undifferentiation, and that the baby is still unable to consistently and clearly distinguish his caregiving objects from himself. What is more important is the fact that, if the baby is to develop a proper sense of reality, the caregiver's near-perfect adaptation to the baby's needs and the baby's attendant experiences of omnipotent control over the object need to be curtailed. Simply put, the baby must be subjected to gradual *disillusionment*. Only then can he come to experience objects as something other and real, and not simply as magically manipulable extensions of himself.

Various environmental scaffoldings support the progression from undifferentiated primary creativity to more realistic and diversified forms of creative interaction. From early on, the caregiver's face functions as a *mirroring* element that assists not only in perceiving oneself as separate, but also in relating to the external world creatively (Winnicott, 1971, pp. 112–118). To clarify what this mirroring entails, Winnicott asks: "What does the baby see when he or she looks at the mother's face?" (p. 112). In terms of objective perception, he simply sees the face as it is: as something that moves, that has certain physical features, and so on. However, when the caregiver is attentively attuned to the baby's occurrent experience and responds accordingly, the face also functions as a mirror: the baby then sees *himself*. In this case, "the mother is looking at the baby and *what she looks like is related to what she sees there*" (p. 112, emphasis in original).

Seeing the caregiver 'looking' like this gives rise to two important experiences in the baby. First, he gradually learns to *trust* in his capacity to elicit affirming reactions from other persons and to exert influence on the external world more generally. Second, responsive mirroring of the baby's experience fosters his capacity for *creative apperception*, namely, the ability to not only perceive what is out there, *objectively*, but also to experience that what is out there can be *subjectively* saturated and meaningfully interlinked with one's own needs, desires, fantasies, etc.

Mirroring cannot, however, be taken for granted. For example, the caregiver's face might predominantly reflect his or her own experience instead of the baby's, or be defensively rigid, avoidant, or blank. When the baby is routinely denied responsive mirroring, objective perception comes to suppress "that which might have been the beginning of a significant exchange with the world, a two-way process in which self-enrichment alternates with the discovery of meaning in the world of seen things" (Winnicott, 1971, p. 113). In other words, if the caregiver's face is unresponsive, "then a mirror is a thing to be looked at but not to be looked into", perceived rather than apperceived (p. 113). If the baby is regularly denied the experience of getting back what he is giving, any budding sense of creative capability is in danger of being cut short. In terms of niche construction, the given dyadic scaffold lacks in both dependability and robust reciprocality.

Winnicott notes that infants react in different ways to such deficiencies. Some do not quite give up hope and do all they can "to see in the object some meaning that ought to be there if only it could be felt" (1971, p. 113). Others study the caregiver's face to forecast his or her moods, and in this way try to discern when it is safe to be needy or spontaneous and when it is better to withdraw from contact. Finally, as mentioned earlier, the baby may submit to looking elsewhere for vital affective mirroring/scaffolding.

Gradually, objects apart from the caregivers begin to figure more prominently in furthering the baby's experiential and creative capacities. This is especially apparent in so-called *transitional phenomena*, which arise at approximately 4 to 12 months of age as infants start to "weave other-than-me objects into the personal pattern" (Winnicott, 1971, pp. 3, 1–25). Characteristically, the baby's autoerotic experiences of thumb-sucking become entangled with other simultaneous activities, such as mouthing and babbling, taking part of a blanket into the mouth with the fingers, caressing and sucking on napkins, etc. At the same time, "thinking, or *fantasying*, gets *linked up* with these functional experiences" (p. 4, my italics). Repeated instances of this kind of imaginative linking open up an intermediate area of experience between thumb and external object; between oral eroticism and true object-relationship; between undifferentiated primary creativity and the projection of fantasy, desire, etc. into external objects (p. 2). Transitional phenomena thus carry the baby from a world in which things are primarily experienced as merged extensions of the self, towards an intermediate area where subjective reality and shared objective reality begin to *co-emerge*, and yet remain experientially *interweaved*.

From within the sphere of transitional phenomena, a specific rag or soft toy will typically emerge and become established as vitally soothing for the baby. This special *transitional object* defends the baby against anxiety by standing in for the nurturer's care in his or her absence, and, in so doing, manifests the rudimentary use of a *symbol* (Winnicott, 1971, p. 96). In this way, it also advances the nascent experience of engaging with things creatively. Importantly, the transitional object is not a hallucination or a mental object, but an actual thing: the individual's first not-me possession. And yet, in the infant's experience, it is not an entirely objective and separate object either. It exists – and in its transitional role can *only* exist – in the intermediate area between subjectivity and objectivity. As Winnicott puts it, the transitional object is located in the "space and time where and when the mother is in transition from being (in the baby's mind) merged in with the infant and alternatively being experienced as an object to be perceived rather than conceived of" (p. 96). Winnicott asks us to accept this paradox and to never challenge the child by asking: "Did you create this object, or did you find it conveniently lying around?" (p. 96). In the middle ground between subjective and objective reality, the baby both creates *and* finds the all-important toy.

This finally brings us to Winnicott's notions of the *potential space* and *playing* (Winnicott, 1971, pp. 38–64, 95–110). To all intents and purposes, the potential space is synonymous with the intermediate area outlined earlier vis-à-vis transitional phenomena. It designates the experiential space "at the interplay between there being nothing but me and there being objects and phenomena outside omnipotent control" (p. 100). As mentioned, the emergence of this space requires dependable nurture and the gradual lowering of the caregivers' adaptation to the baby's needs. If the baby is given the chance to exist creatively through good enough care, he will develop the extended ability "to use actual objects to be creative into and with", that is, to engage with them creatively (p. 101). In slightly different terms, a space emerges which can be creatively filled in by *playing*. Winnicott states that in playing, and perhaps only in playing, is the individual free to be creative (p. 53). He also maintains that later cultural experience is rooted in the creativity that is first manifested in early play (p. 100). As he explains it,

> the baby's confidence in the mother's reliability, and therefore in that of other people and things, makes possible a separating-out of the not-me from the me. At the same time, however, it can be said that separation is avoided by the filling in of the potential space with creative playing, with the use of symbols, and with all that eventually adds up to a cultural life.
>
> (p. 109)

In short, the potential space comes to serve as the trusted basis and 'location' for all playing, creative activity, and cultural experience.

To be clear, the potential space is not some kind of psychological entity that exists separately from or prior to the subject's interaction with objects – it is not a 'place in' or 'part of' the mind, as it were. Instead, it designates a relationally constituted *mode of experiencing* where subjective and objective realities intermix and are accentuated in qualitatively varying ways. On one end of the continuum, experience is dominated by personal fantasies, wishes, dreams, and the like; in this case, any given object is, in essence, "a bundle of projections" (Winnicott, 1971, p. 88). On the other end, objects are experienced as strictly separate and autonomous: as factual elements of the world that must be rigidly conformed to and accepted as they are. To clarify these distinctions, Winnicott notes how schizoid individuals tend to be out of touch with shared reality and prone to delusion and hallucination, while others may be "so firmly anchored in objectively perceived reality that they are ill in the opposite direction of being out of touch with the subjective world and with the creative approach to fact" (pp. 66–67). Even so, Winnicott sees no sharp line between health and illness in this respect. The accentuation of subjective and objective reality can fluctuate considerably in the changing situations and contexts of everyday living.

That being said, we all tend to 'inhabit' the potential space in our own relatively set and idiosyncratic ways. In this connection, Winnicott speaks of the "fate" of the potential space; it may or may not, for instance, become a "vital area" of one's experiential world (1971, p. 101, pp. 106–108). Varied individual fates are in large part due to differing life experiences. In unfavorable circumstances, the baby is not granted a space in which to play, or this space is severely constricted or highly precarious. The expected psychological outcome of this is an impoverished capacity for generating meaningful symbols and experiencing shared cultural living (p. 102). Total deprivation is, however, rare: a minimal creative impulse or creative capacity can be found in nearly everyone and can, to different extents, be restored and cultivated throughout life (pp. 68–69). From this point of view, what is most interesting is the distinctive manner in which the potential space actually *functions* in any given individual's experiential world, for instance, with respect to its expansion versus diminution, its vitality versus frailty, its diversity versus uniformity, and its overall dynamics of accentuation.

Let us pause here to summarize Winnicott's developmental account of creativity within a niche construction/scaffolding framework. For the infant, there is no stable distinction of me and not-me in the earliest developmental niche. The baby's primary caregivers both uphold this experience and foster its eventual transformation into a more differentiated sense of reality. Caregiving is initially geared towards providing what the baby is ready to find via near-perfect adaptation to his needs. This enables the baby to experience primary creativity and illusory control over the caregiving object. Soon, by way of responsive mirroring, transitional phenomena, and gradual disillusionment, the baby not only begins to distinguish between himself and the world, but also gains a rudimentary capacity for creative apperception and symbolization. During this process, the baby usually adopts a particular non-caregiver object – a transitional object – to keep his separation anxiety in check. For a while, this special object serves as an indispensable affective scaffold for the baby. Moreover, its use manifests the individual's first properly creative engagement with a material environmental resource, and in this way initiates the transition from a limited, caregiver-centered niche towards niches in which an increasing number of other resources are found/created to enable, support, and modify personal experience. This overall developmental shift depends in turn on the emergence of the potential space, wherein subjective psychic reality and active manipulation of the objective world commingle in play. Finally, over time, playing and creative relating begin to take on more sophisticated and culturally shared forms. Slowly but surely, niche construction expands, diversifies, and becomes experientially more enriching. In sum, if all goes well, early affective scaffolding will instill in the individual a basic confidence that the world can be engaged with creatively.

From creative relating to artistic creativity and painting

As mentioned, Winnicott was more interested in the preconditions of common creative living than in specialized forms of creative activity. Even so, his writings do contain some thought-provoking remarks about *artistic* creativity as well. He explicitly distinguishes his approach from models of creativity that accentuate the innate aggressive fantasies of the baby and the subsequent reparation of destroyed inner objects through artistic work (here Winnicott refers specifically to Melanie Klein's thinking) (1971, pp. 69–71). He also distances himself from psychoanalytical aesthetic studies that scrutinize the interconnections between artistic works and their creators' instinctually driven developmental histories – as exemplified by Freud's essay on Leonardo da Vinci (1910). Such analyses, Winnicott claims, only tend to "irritate artists and creative people in general", and lose sight of the main theme of interest, namely, the "creative impulse itself" (p. 69). In this way, Winnicott makes it clear that he finds it problematic to emphasize hereditary instinctual drive over environmental provision. He states outright that, by taking "refuge in heredity", both Freud and Klein "avoided . . . the full implication of dependence and therefore of the environmental factor" (1971, pp. 70–71). A proper account of (artistic) creativity thus calls for a fuller understanding of the environmental context in which it develops and unfolds.

Winnicott also sees a critical link between creativity and *self-discovery*, by which he means the achievement of a unitary sense of "I AM, I am alive, I am myself" (1971, pp. 53–64). On this view, creative living is much more than merely existing; "it is finding a way to exist as oneself, and to relate to objects as oneself, and to have a self into which to retreat for relaxation" (p. 117). The search for the self can be successful only if the environment can be trusted to reflect back in personally meaningful form previously unstructured and shapeless aspects of one's experience. This interchange presupposes, in both childhood and adulthood, an area where one can relax and play in a non-purposive way, and out of which creative reaching-out and form-giving can proceed (p. 55). In other words, it is only in the potential space "that the individual child or adult is able to be creative and to use the whole personality, and it is *only in creativity that the individual discovers the self*" (p. 54, my italics).

In this connection Winnicott makes a rather intriguing comment about artistic activity:

> In a search for the self the person concerned may have produced something valuable in terms of art, but a successful artist may be universally acclaimed and yet have failed to find the self that he or she is looking for. The self is not really to be found in what is made out of products of the body or mind, however valuable these constructs may be in terms of beauty, skill, and impact. If the artist (in whatever medium) is searching for the self, then it can be said that in all probability there is already some failure for that artist in the field of general creative living. The finished creation never heals the underlying lack of a sense of self.
>
> (1971, pp. 54–55)

Winnicott seems to be doing two things here. On the one hand, he is making a categorical claim about the insufficiency of artistic creations for repairing a substantially impaired sense of self. On the other, he is describing the kind of artistic activity that may nonetheless stem from such an underlying deficiency. Indeed, Winnicott presents the cited passage in a *clinically* oriented context, namely, with regard to patients "who are trying to find themselves in the products of their creative experiences" (1971, p. 54). This supports the interpretation that, due to shortcomings in their early caretaking niches, *some* individuals are exceedingly driven to create for themselves compensatory affective scaffolds through artistic work. In other words, owing to ontogenetically instigated "failures in the field of creative living", certain individuals are strongly motivated to construct, through art, surrogate mirrors that support their basic self-experience (for elaborations of this idea, see, e.g., Fuller, 1980; Wright, 2009). For all that, Winnicott also suggests that an extensively frail, fractured, or disorganized sense of self can never be fully or permanently consolidated via artistic work alone.

Regarding mirroring and its vicissitudes, Winnicott mentions Francis Bacon as an artist whose distorted painted visages evince a strong concern for the face, and for seeing and being seen. Although Winnicott admits to knowing nothing of the painter's private life, he suggests that, in his work, Bacon "is seeing himself in his mother's face, but with some twist in him or her that maddens both him and us" (1971, p. 114). He adds that in this looking, Bacon seems "to be painfully striving towards being seen" (p. 114). If we choose to view Bacon and his artwork through this interpretive lens, he may indeed strike us as the kind of individual who persistently searches for himself in the mirror of his own creative products; yet, since he can never fully find himself there, has to keep on painting/looking.

Despite these somewhat bleak observations, I do not take Winnicott to suggest that artistic creativity is necessarily driven by serious deficiencies in early mirroring or caretaking. It would also be in stark contrast to the spirit of his overall outlook to maintain that artistic creativity – as a specific manifestation of creative living – cannot appreciably enhance self-experience. Indeed, in a letter to Victor Smirnoff, a child psychoanalyst who was in the process of translating his *Transitional Objects and Transitional Phenomena* (1953) into French, Winnicott suggests that artistic creativity can be a means for the artist to *feel real*, and sometimes even the *only* means to do so:

> Here I am trying in my summary to relate experiencing to the transitional phenomena. I am implying that actual experiencing does not stem directly either from the individual's psychic reality nor from the individual's external relationships. This sounds rather startling but you can perhaps get my meaning if you think of a Van Gogh experiencing, that is to say, feeling real, when painting one of his pictures, but feeling unreal in his relationships with external reality and in his private withdrawn inner life. I think that this idea badly needs working out but it is this sort of thing that I am trying to convey.
>
> (in Rodman, 1987, p. 124)

Elsewhere, Winnicott points out that artists also enable their *audiences* to feel real and alive when life threatens to become too overbearing (1965, p. 47).

On a final note, Winnicott makes a broad connection between artistic creativity and transitional phenomena. He discusses how the child's transitional object eventually loses its psychic import, and is thence "not so much forgotten as relegated to limbo" (1971, p. 5). This psychological shift happens as creative symbolization begins to spread out over the cultural field. Indeed, Winnicott suggests that at this point the subject of transitional phenomena "widens out into that of play, and of artistic creativity and appreciation, and of religious feeling", etc. (p. 5). On these grounds, we may conjecture that, like the early transitional object, the work of art is both actual and symbolic; that it is shaped by the subject to contain her needs, desires, and fantasies; that it comes to have a vitality and reality of its own; and that it enables one to 'inhabit', in an exceptionally vivid and absorbed manner, the experiential area where subjective and objective coincide (see also Spitz, 1985, p. 146).

Perhaps Winnicott's view of artistic creativity can be encapsulated as follows. Most people develop at least a rudimentary capacity for creative apperception, play, and symbolization through good enough early care. These capacities become individually actualized in the (artistic) cultural field to greater or lesser degrees and in various different ways. More importantly, however, and regardless of individual variation in creative ability, every human being is ineluctably faced with the task of establishing and sustaining a vital, meaningful, and cohesive sense of self. Each person, and hence each artist, engages in this perpetual process within the potential space and its individually evolved – and evolv*ing* – experiential parameters. From this point of view, artistic creativity is a specialized and advanced form of creative living, and one through which the self may be enlivened, unified, and made more real.

This is basically where Winnicott leaves us with regard to artistic creativity, and it has thus been left to others to fill in the picture. Fortunately, many writers have applied, developed, and/or critiqued Winnicott's ideas with a perceptive eye on art (see Fuller, 1980; Rose, 1980; Spitz, 1985; Bollas, 1999; Hagman, 2005; Sayers, 2007; Townsend, 2019). I will next focus on one such contribution, namely that of Kenneth Wright (2009), in order to help spell out my own Winnicott-based approach to painting and painterly affectivity.

True to Winnicott, Wright regards transitional phenomena and maternal mirroring as the developmental cornerstones for later artistic creativity, including painting. In his view, the finding and creating of the transitional object initiates "a line of development in which external objects can be invested with personal significance rather than simply accepted as they are" (Wright, 2009, p. 142). Wright describes this creative investment as a type of commerce: we learn to put ourselves *into* objects in order to realize ourselves *through* them. The development of this capacity also requires sufficient mirroring. In Wright's terms, the caregiver's face functions as a *responsive medium* from which the baby can draw out the *significant forms* of his own experience, meaning those forms that are suitably consonant with his occurrent affective state (pp. 142–145). In similar fashion, the artist seeks in her art the kinds of forms that reflect her subjective experience with satisfactory accuracy. Hence, on Wright's Winnicottian account, both artistic creativity and early dyadic interaction involve (a) an emotional reaching-out by the subject towards the object, with the expectation of a response; (b) a medium that allows itself to be transformed; and (c) a finding of forms within that medium that simultaneously reveal and actualize one's inner experience (p. 144).

Wright points out that the artist has more *control* over her artistic creation than the infant does over his caregiver. The painter can modify the painting until it gives back the responses that she is looking for, perhaps even more reliably than her caregivers have done during infancy (2009, pp. 144–145). Wright thus regards artistic creativity as an activity that can compensate for earlier deficiencies in provision. It enables, on a more mature level, the resumption and revival of an unfinished and possibly insufficient process of mirroring. In this way, painting can come to serve a therapeutic function. Wright summarizes this stance as follows:

> The artist, we could say, operates in dialogue with his canvas, and creates an illusory and expressive surface through his technique. With all the varied elements of that technique, he learns to draw from his medium forms that reflect and recreate the pulse and rhythm of his inner life. According to this view, the new relation between artist and medium parallels, but also improves on, an earlier preverbal relation with the mother, whose facial expressions mirrored, or failed to mirror, the emotional gestures of the artist as infant.
>
> (2009, p. 145)

As much as Wright underlines the importance of mirroring, he wants to avoid overemphasizing the role of the face alone, especially at the expense of other bodily aspects of caregiving. He thus turns to Daniel Stern's (1985) concept of *attunement* to develop a more comprehensive account of what goes on between infant and caregiver and, accordingly, between painter and painting. In Stern's theory, attunement consists in a *recasting* of the infant's subjective state by its caregivers. This means that the caregiver responds to the shapes, rhythms, contours, etc. of the infant's experience as revealed in his behavior. Crucially, the caregiver does not mimic the infant – sound for sound, movement for movement – but instead varies and transforms elements of the baby's experience into idiosyncratic expressive patterns, often cross-modally (for example, from motion to sound). As a result, the infant can inhabit the reasonably accurate forms provided by the caregiver, thrive in the shared space of attunement, and feel enhanced by feelings of resonance. As expected, Wright considers such early bodily attunement as a precursor to the dynamics of artistic creativity:

> Looking towards the later transformations of art, it could be said that in passing through the *medium* of the mother, the baby's lived emotional pattern is creatively changed and begins to confront him as an objective form in the gestures which the mother has "shaped".
>
> (p. 147)

The art object thus recasts the experience of the artist and gives it back to her in personally resonant form (p. 146). By treating the canvas as a "surrogate maternal extension", the painter takes over the caregivers' form-making capacity and brings it to fruition in her work (pp. 147, 152).

On this distinctly Winnicottian account, then, "*finding oneself in, and through, an objective medium* is central to understanding the artistic enterprise" (Wright, 2009, p. 143, emphasis in original). In infancy, mirroring and attunement "literally bring the self into being", and these very same processes are subsequently needed to support the experience of "going on being" (p. 153). Without proper environmental attunement, disparate elements of subjective experience cannot be organized into larger, coherent patterns, and are therefore unavailable for self-integration and self-enrichment. Hence, "the artist's pressing need is to bring his own self into being through his creative work", and it is only those creations that resonate with his experiential world that effectively enable him to "exist and feel real" (pp. 153–154). In this way, artistic creativity aims for the unity and wholeness of the self.

In general, I find this type of developmental approach compelling, and adopt it as my basic theoretical framework. That said, it does have its potential pitfalls. One possible risk in linking adult art-making to infantile interaction is to misconstrue the significance of *occurrent* affective experience. Early dyadic attunement may indeed hinge on the infant's ongoing affective states. What the baby is feeling at the given moment is what needs to be recast and mirrored in satisfactory form by the caregiver. However, transposing this dynamic to painters' interactions with their paintings is a more contentious move. Arguably, whatever the artist is feeling *during* the creative process is not necessarily or even commonly the main 'target' of aesthetic-creative formalization, realization, or mirroring. While there are artistic traditions that encourage painters to articulate their here-and-now affective experience into paint, this cannot be said to apply to the practice of painting in toto. Simply put, painters often seek form for something *beyond* or *other than* their ongoing feelings.

This raises a more general question about the nature and role of affectivity in artistic creativity. When Wright discusses an amalgam of "subjective feeling states", "human feeling and experience", the "lived emotional pattern", the "emotional self", and "latent elements of affective life" as *that which is mirrored back* in painting, he is clearly placing great emphasis on all things affective (2009, pp. 145–153). However, such accentuation risks overlooking the fact that adult creativity is equally based on sophisticated capacities to think conceptually and analytically; to generate complex ideas, plans, and narratives; to imagine things and to also manipulate these things in imagination; to recognize and attend to the social, cultural, and historical aspects of one's creations; to make evaluative aesthetic judgments; to spin elaborate fantasies; to reminisce in detail; and so on. Simply put, mature mental life is not affective in the same predominant, all-embracing, and disorganized way that infantile experience is. Rather, it is an advanced complex of cognitive, affective, and conative faculties.

I therefore maintain that artistic creation need not primarily concern or target the (formless) *affective* elements of experience. Again, some painting praxes might seek to bypass cognition in order to reach the raw affective realm, as it were. However, the artist may also attempt to articulate, for example, carefully considered political, religious, or philosophical ideas; complex imaginings and fantasies; specific memories, situations, and events; current perceptions of the environment; or, more often than not, different combinations of these. Of course, such endeavors will inevitably involve feeling, too. However, acknowledging this is altogether different from suggesting that affective experience is that which is primarily or ultimately targeted and materialized in artistic creation. For this reason, I do not find it productive to tie painterly creativity too exclusively to expressing or actualizing the 'emotional self'. In more general ontogenetic terms, we should be cautious not to overstress early affective experience at the expense of maturity and the individual's overall mental capacities (see Fonagy & Target, 2003, p. 20).

On a related precautionary note, when we *do* opt to link together infantile and mature forms of interaction, we should be aware of the difference between relations of *influence* and relations of *similarity*. Consider the following observation from Wright: "[T]he canvas surface in painting is a *derivative*, or *analogue*, of the mother's expressive face in infancy, and functions in a similar way: as a responsive and mirroring extension of the self" (2009, p. 13, my italics). This statement might strike us as somewhat ambivalent in that it seems to blend together two different claims. On the one hand, the term 'derivative' suggests that early interaction has a relevant *effect* on the later activity of painting. That is to say, it indicates that the way the artist relates to her canvas originates in and continues to be based on the way she formerly engaged with her caregivers. This type of proposition is exemplified by the already familiar claim that, in and through painting, the artist seeks to compensate for preceding deficiencies in mirroring and attunement. In this example, early interaction is taken to have a distinctly *motivational* influence, insofar as the artist is driven to paint because of shortcomings in her primary caregiving niche.

On the other hand, the term 'analogue' signifies that early dyadic interaction and painterly creativity are merely *comparable* events or processes. It indicates that they have something noteworthy in common, sharing, for example, experiential, motivational, structural, and/or functional resemblances – the last of which is implied, for instance, by Wright, when he notes that the painting 'functions in a similar way' to the mother's face. Similarity does not, however, necessitate that one of the two compared phenomena derives from the other. Like the early maternal face, the painted canvas may indeed function as a responsive medium and feel like one, too; but these parallels do not yet establish that the later type of responsivity derives from the earlier in any cogent or non-trivial sense. Having said that, similarity and influence do not necessarily exclude each other, either, and can therefore both apply to the relation between painting and early development. The takeaway point is this: if we choose to analyze the nature of painterly creativity by linking together aspects of infancy and adulthood, we should distinguish between influence and similarity. This should also help us to avoid any tenuous or reductive tracing of mature processes and experiences to specific earlier developmental phases and interactions.

With these considerations in mind, and in line with Wright and other Winnicottian theorists, I regard painting as an activity that takes place in the potential space. It unfolds in the intermediate area of experience wherein subjective reality and active manipulation of the objective world coincide and commingle in creative play. As outlined earlier, the vital functioning of the potential space presupposes confidence in one's own creative capacities. This trust is established via good enough primary caregiving and is eventually extended to cover other people, things, and activities. In this way, the *basic preconditions* for engaging creatively with the world – and hence, for creating paintings – are laid down in early interaction.

What's more, *how* the potential space comes to be idiosyncratically 'filled in' and 'inhabited' also begins to develop in the early caretaking niche. Differences in provision, trust, disillusionment, and affective scaffolding contribute to individual variation in how expansive or restricted, vital or frail, rich or scarce this space is experienced to be. Different ontogenetic paths also lead to divergent ways of accentuating and intermixing subjective and objective reality. On these grounds, the 'fate' of the potential space will arguably also affect how any individual painter relates to her own creations and experiences the creative process more generally. For example, some artists' creative work may be abundantly suffused with subjective fantasies, desires, and wishes. Others may in turn comply more closely with the demands and standards of a shared, objective reality. On this account, then, painting unfolds in a potential space whose functioning and experiential parameters derive in a relevant way from earlier interactions.

To add to these relatively standard Winnicottian insights, I submit that painting does not merely rest on and occur in the potential space. It also enables the artist to engage with various concerns that are woven into the experiential fabric of that very same space. This proposition can be broken down as follows. As discussed, the newborn has no stable sense of what is me and not-me. It is only through gradual disillusionment that he begins to recognize the independent existence of things. This process does not, however, carve reality simply into two distinct opposites of self and world. It also establishes the third, intermediate area of experience, namely, the potential space. And this brings us to the crux of the matter. The *emergence of the potential space gives rise to various experiential issues that matter deeply to one's being*, or, more precisely, to how one relates to oneself, others, and things, and to situations, events, and states of affairs. First and foremost, once the potential space – as a mode of experience – is established, the individual cannot but be perennially concerned with how subjective and objective realities intermingle in his own being. Winnicott attests to the same phenomenon when he states that "no human being is free from the strain of relating inner and outer reality" (1971, p. 13). To all intents and purposes, the "task of reality-acceptance is never completed" (p. 13).

I designate these basic 'strains' and 'tasks' of human existence as *core existential concerns*. Simply put, they are concerns that fundamentally and perpetually bear upon our being in the world. Gilbert Rose illuminates this existential necessity aptly with the concept of "transitional process" (1980, p. 112–129). In his Winnicottian view, the self (organism) is an open system that develops mutually with its environment. The dynamic equilibrium sought and maintained between a relatively fluid self and an objective reality is not limited to the transitional phenomena of childhood but is a process that continues into adulthood. Thus, there is an ongoing transitional interplay between self and reality: a confluence of self-centered and object-centered interests (pp. 112–114). All of this unfolds on a continuum of creative imagination and adaptation to the 'real' world. In sum, 'transitional process' signifies the continuous workings of the self in mixing together elements of subjective and objective reality in the potential space.

In addition to the basic task of relating *subjective* and *objective reality*, various further existential concerns are integral to the potential space. For instance, we must continuously negotiate and demarcate *what is self* and *what is not-self.* In coping with the fact of our separate existence and possible isolation, we must also address the attendant need of *connecting with others* in ways that enable us to be affirmatively seen and recognized. A further, closely related concern centers on the need to achieve a *sense of vitality* – that is, of feeling fully alive. Fundamentally, what we need and desire most is "to feel that life is real, to find life worth living" (Winnicott, 1971, p. 98). The flipside of this is a sense of utter futility and meaninglessness, even deadness. In my account, then, the potential space is home to various concerns that continuously press upon our being. At the same time, it is the area where we can play and relax, and from which creative apperception and form-giving can proceed. As such, the potential space enables us to engage with our existential concerns creatively.

Viewed in this light, artistic creativity is a kind of existential play *with* and *within* the potential space. And this is why painting, too, can become so important. The painter creates for herself a *transformative affective scaffold*: a crucial means for dealing with core existential concerns, for experiencing the playful and productive interweaving of subjective and objective realities and, ultimately, for transforming her basic sense of being. Indeed, some of the most intense and pleasurable feelings in painting are inextricably bound up with concerns about subjective versus objective, me versus not-me, separateness versus connection, and vitality versus psychic sterility. In other words, painting can scaffold beneficial feelings of fluidity, merger, unity, contact, resonance, aliveness, transcendence, and the like. Painters come to value and desire these kinds of affective states because they galvanize, enrich, and (re)structure their overall sense of existence. The remainder of the book will be dedicated to the demonstration and further elaboration of these ideas.

Concluding remarks

Before moving on, however, two final remarks about my overall theoretical approach are in order. First, although I have focused exclusively on dyadic interaction, I do not mean to suggest that other elements of the early developmental niche are less important or insignificant in the development of creativity. I have chosen the specific, narrower scope of investigation to achieve a relatively thorough examination of one pivotal aspect of the caretaking niche. This has enabled me to discuss in detail how dyadic interaction fosters a basic sense of trust, contributes to the emergence of a creative world-relation, and establishes several core existential concerns that continue to inform later painterly creativity and affectivity.

Second, it is worth noting that many psychoanalytical models of artistic creativity, including Wright's, presuppose that first there is something affective *in* the subject, typically in a formless or latent state, which is then *projected* into the outer art object, worked on, and eventually mirrored back and *reintegrated* into the self in altered, meaningful form. I find that such 'inner-outer commerce' tells only part of the affective story of painting. To fill in the story, I extend the spotlight from the expressive articulation of inner affective states to the *evocation* of affects which cannot be said to exist, even formlessly, prior to the painterly interaction, and which are essentially made possible and supported by the activity of painting itself. Simply put, I aim to analyze the co-constitution of novel and desirable affects in the interaction between painter and painting. This suggests that, by way of painting, the artist seeks to feel things that are not in any sense inside her, merely waiting to be given form and realized. Experientially speaking, painting can thus be taken to deal with what goes on in the potential space – in the dynamic association of subjective and objective – rather than with any preexisting inner affective states.

Chapter 4

Vitality

Many painters experience their artworks as living things, portraying them as 'partners' or 'beings' that respond to their painterly gestures, propose further courses of action, and sometimes even take over the creative effort. Artists accordingly talk about surrendering to their paintings and conversing with them to hear what they have to say. Moreover, if a painting is properly nurtured it is said to breathe and to grow, but if things go awry, it will suffocate and perhaps even be worked to death. Painter Olli Piippo describes these animistic aspects of painting vividly:

> My paintings become creature-like as my work progresses. Each painting grows to be an individual: a developing and breathing body that can't be forced under control or any predetermined intentions. It is therefore more productive to surrender to the thought processes offered by the painting and to accept that the final product will be something other than initially planned. Only by listening sensitively to one's paintings can the right kind of feeling be found. In this sense, I see my paintings as collaborators.
>
> (Personal interview; see also Saarinen, 2019)

Juhana Blomstedt has also referred to his paintings as partners-in-dialogue. "I relate to the painting as another person with whom I converse", he confirms. At the outset,

> there is nothing but a helpless mark on the canvas. It's like a child trying to utter its first word. . . . Then the canvas begins to demand that, since you've already done this to me, you must next do this and then do that.
>
> (Jäämeri, 2007, my translation)

Blomstedt explains that the dialogue continues until neither has anything left to say to the other. "That's when the painting is finished" (Jäämeri, 2007, my translation). Finally, Susanne Gottberg portrays the essence of her painting as follows:

> Even if a space seems empty, it always has a sense of presence. I paint in order to discover that distinct presence – and when I find it, it awakens a feeling that I am in dialogue with a living thing.
>
> (*The Third Factor* exhibition text, Kunsthalle Helsinki, 1 June to 4 August, 2019)

Obviously, these painters are not delusional – they know full well that their paintings are not *really* alive. Accordingly, one might contend that animistic depictions of art-making are always just metaphorical: nothing but figures of speech that only the naïve would regard as literal accounts of experience. There is undoubtedly a good deal of metaphorical parlance in play here. However, I do not believe that a strictly figurative interpretation can adequately capture the experiential truth of the matter. Instead, I maintain that some artists *do* indeed feel their paintings-in-progress to be alive, albeit in ways that are peculiar to painterly creativity.

More precisely, I submit that there are two varyingly actualized and emphasized aspects to experiencing paintings as living objects. First, and more simply, they can be experienced as *organic* things, that is, as things that possess certain attributes of living matter, such as the ability to grow, to change, and to develop. Second, paintings may moreover be experienced as *agentive* organic things, namely, as responsive, interactive, communicative, and/or autonomous contributors to the creative process. As such, they are typically sensed to open up novel opportunities, to prompt certain painterly reactions, and, in some cases, to even come into being of their own accord. This means that artists may experience their paintings to be organically alive without experiencing them to be agentive; the latter feature, when co-present with the former, amounts to a richer and more advanced sense of the aliveness of paintings.

To elaborate on this basic proposition, I identify three sets of factors that contribute to the aliveness of paintings. First, I discuss the role of *cultural* and *discursive* factors in supporting animistic and anthropomorphic notions of painting. In other words, I consider the ways in which extant conceptions and discourses concerning artistry foster the experience of paintings as living/agentive beings. After that, I shift to the *psychological* and *developmental* factors that support the given feelings. I focus specifically on artists' vitalistic fantasies and expectations, and examine how these underlying, mostly unconscious factors are rooted in early dyadic interactions. Third, I call attention to some of the *material* and *metamorphic* factors that account for the aliveness of paintings. That is to say, I pinpoint some of the tactile and visual qualities of paint that contribute to the vital appearance of paintings. Along with this, I illuminate how the transformation of paintings during the creative process makes them more liable to be experienced as living things. To conclude the chapter on a distinctly existential note, I suggest that the aliveness of one's paintings also enables *oneself* to feel more alive and connected. In this manner, the given feelings satisfy a core existential striving for meaningful and enriching contacts with the surrounding world. And, for this reason, vitalistic feelings are deemed by many artists to be especially valuable and desirable.

It's alive! From Pygmalion to present-day painters

I have pointed out that professional painting is always *diachronically* scaffolded (see Chapter 2). It is a practice that is necessarily structured by existing aesthetic styles and traditions, by long-running discourses about painting and creativity, and by established artistic conventions, ideologies, and norms. Crucially, these and many other diachronically operating scaffolds influence how painters experience their own painterly praxes, even if the painters themselves are not fully aware of this link. Simply put, painters paint in historical and cultural contexts that enable, support, and make intelligible certain kinds of (affective) relations to their paintings.

Feeling one's paintings to be alive is no exception to this rule. Indeed, the notion of artworks as living 'others' has a lengthy history in our shared imagination. One of its earliest manifestations can be found in the eighth-century myth of Pygmalion and Galatea (from Ovid's *Metamorphoses*). Besides being king of Cyprus, Pygmalion was a sculptor who carved for himself a beautiful female figure out of ivory. Having named the woman/statue Galatea, Pygmalion began to treat her as if she were a real person and, soon enough, fell in love with her. His desire for Galatea grew so intense that, upon visiting the altar of Aphrodite, he prayed for a living bride just like her. When Pygmalion returned home, he kissed Galatea and found her lips to be warm and her 'skin' to be soft. His wish had been fulfilled.

The Pygmalion myth embodies the basic trope of the artist being so enthralled by his own creation that he begins to regard it as a living thing or, more precisely, as another person. This powerful and long-standing theme has taken on various forms in Western art. Art historian Isabelle Graw asks us to consider, for example, allegorical depictions from the sixteenth century in which painting appears as a female figure that seduces the painter, who, in turn, is always portrayed as male and fully devoted to her service. In short, in these depictions "painting was imagined as a male procreative act from which women artists were excluded" (Graw, 2018, p. 337). As Graw points out, we can find further variations of this trope in nineteenth-century novels about artists, for instance in Honoré de Balzac's *Le Chef-d'œuvre inconnu* (1831) and Émile Zola's *L'œuvre* (1886). She notes how in these novels,

> not only did the painter render and the viewer perceive the subject of a painting as brimming with life, but the painting itself mutated into a quasi-human (always female) entity, a being making relentless demands of its creator and abiding no rivals.
>
> (2018, p. 24)

Putting aside the blatant chauvinism of these cases, they attest to the power of a deeper "vitalistic fantasy": a fantasy in which human attributes such as will and self-command are projected into lifeless objects (p. 24). This basic fantasy has continued to resurface in modified form to this very day in the production, subject matter, and reception of art. In fact, Graw goes as far as to say that it is "a leitmotif that runs through *all* painting discourses" (p. 55, my italics).

It is beyond the scope of this study to elaborate further on the numerous discourses and practices that have reinforced the trope of living and agentive paintings. It is, however, worth noting that artists too have done their share in upholding the myth. Graw discusses Sigmar Polke, Albert Oehlen, and Charline von Heyl, for instance, as present-day painters who "have tended to stylize painting into a quasi-subjective entity that confronts the painter with specific demands", and who have accordingly critiqued, ironized, and/or played with this notion in their own artwork (2018, p. 56). To add to this, Graw suggests that the vitalistic trope has manifested in a somewhat different way in the work of so-called anti-subjectivist painters. By delegating issues of pictorial composition to outside sources and by applying mechanized and random production methods to execute their work, these painters have deliberately sought to "negate the artist's hand" and to thus "efface themselves from the productive process" (p. 116; see also pp. 88–106). In Graw's perception, many of the paintings created in this manner – for example, by Ellsworth Kelly and Gerhard Richter – invoke a surprisingly strong sense of "the pictures' self-agency", and, owing to this, have consolidated "the modern myth of the self-creating picture" (p. 116). In sum, then, painters can be said to have upheld the trope of paintings as living agentic things in at least three different ways: first, by portraying their own painterly experience in animistic terms; second, by incorporating the vitalistic trope into the subject matter of their own artworks; and third, by imparting to their paintings a distinct air of autonomy and self-sufficiency. By doing these things, painters have also reinforced the culturally sustained scaffolds that influence *other* artists' experiences of creativity, as well.

For all its cultural-discursive embeddedness, I maintain that the notion of paintings as living things is essentially grounded in the actual *experience* of creativity or, rather, in hundreds of years of collectively accumulated and shared experiences of art-making. I think that this common experiential basis also accounts for the power and persistence of the trope. It is something that many painters can relate to, as they recognize its truth vis-à-vis their own painterly practice. Graw arrives at more or less the same conclusion:

> We might brand these manifold attempts to anthropomorphize paintings as a return of superstition, animism, and magic, and we would not be entirely wrong. Works of art, after all, are dead matter and not living beings. At the same time, these strategies painters adopt do capture an experience that virtually anyone who produces art has had at one time or another. Whether we write a text or paint a picture – sometimes it seems to us as though the work in our hands were almost producing itself, pushing us forward, raising specific demands. Myth and the experience of production are closely interwoven in the trope of the living picture.
>
> (2018, p. 56)

I will now leave aside myth and trope to examine how the experience of production incorporates vitalistic fantasy. I take as my starting point Graw's intriguing observation that the fantasy of aliveness is tied to "the vitalistic *potential* of painting itself" (2018, p. 24, my italics). What is this vitalistic potential and how, specifically, is it present in painting? My answer to this question will come in two parts. First, I analyze how the relational roots and psychological dynamics of painting contribute to the vitalistic potential at stake, and thus make feelings of aliveness more liable to occur. Then, in the next section, I detail some of the distinctive material and metamorphic features of paintings which give rise to the very same effects.

The relational and psychological dynamics of vitalistic fantasy

Our very first creative experiences arise in relation to other living beings. More than that: it is *only* in relation to other persons that we achieve the ability to be creative at all. Indeed, I have argued that early infant–caregiver interactions instill in the individual the basic capacity and confidence to engage creatively with the world. I have also outlined how this initial creativity gradually diversifies and extends to encompass a wide variety of objects, including artworks (see Chapter 3). For this line of thinking to hold credence, we must presuppose that our experience is inherently *cumulative* and *sedimented.* Philosopher Joona Taipale expresses this presupposition concisely when he writes:

> By becoming something past, experiences do not vanish without a trace. Instead, they invest subjectivity with beliefs, preconceptions, and tendencies that, again, shape the course of our further experiences and even predetermine them to some extent. Each of our experiences carries something from our previous experiences, and in this sense refers back to them, whereas these prior experiences again contain references to the ones preceding them – and so on.
>
> (Taipale, 2014, p. 242)

Needless to say, this notion is fundamental to all psychoanalytical thinking on ontogenesis. To rephrase the gist of it in specifically relational terms, ongoing adult experience is inevitably and unconsciously conditioned by a long personal history of relating with 'objects' – first with those that are present in our caretaking environment, and then more generally with an increasing number of other beings and things. On these grounds, we have good reason to assume that mature art-making will likewise carry experiential traces of earlier, more rudimentary creative interactions, even if the artist is not explicitly aware of this connection.

From this developmental standpoint, I wish to stress that being creative is indelibly stamped with a sense of relating to *animate* objects. As psychoanalyst Marion Milner encapsulates it, the first relationship with the external world is primarily a relationship of one person to another, and only gradually becomes more clearly differentiated into relations with living beings and relations with inanimate things (Milner, 1957, p. 116). To put this in a broader context, we might say that one's world is initially constituted by a predominantly animate caregiving environment, elements of which remain latent in later, mature experience. Indeed, relying on this very notion, Milner points out the "possibility that the adult painter could be basically, even though unconsciously, concerned with an animistically conceived world" (p. 116). That being so,

> the problem of the relation between the painter and his world . . . [is] basically a problem of one's own need and the needs of the "other", a problem of reciprocity between "you" and "me"; with "you" and "me" meaning originally mother and child.
>
> (p. 116)

Thus, owing to the primary developmental conditions of creative experience, and to the sedimentation of such experience, we acquire an unconscious propensity to engage with objects of our own creation as if they were living, responsive, and agentic beings. To be absolutely clear, this vitalistic fantasy is a *potentiality* rather than a manifest feature of all creative actions and situations – and therefore requires certain conditions to be met if it is to be triggered.

Once in effect, vitalistic fantasy also entails various *expectations* which, if fulfilled, reinforce the feeling of the painting's aliveness. Like the fantasy itself, these expectations are rooted in primary infant–caregiver interactions and tend to operate outside conscious awareness. To recap, in passing through the medium of the caregiver, the baby's experience is articulated in external form. Moreover, it is through these engagements that we learn to *anticipate* that (some) external objects will respond to our actions affirmatively and provide our experience with appropriate and satisfying form. This trust-based anticipatory dynamic is cemented into the core of creative interaction and latently carried over to later artistic activity. Thus, when the vitalistic fantasy is rekindled and the painter engages with her painting, she expects it to be receptive and malleable, to be responsive to her actions and gestures, and to provide satisfactory form to elements of her own experience (see Chapters 3 and 6). On an unconscious level, the artist relates to the artwork as a 'surrogate caregiver' and accordingly projects onto it some of the caregivers' vital qualities and agentic capacities. That being so, the artist will expect the painting to 'behave' in analogous, animate ways, and when it does, the sense of its aliveness will only be intensified.

To illuminate this peculiar experience, let us return to the theme of *dialogue*. As art historian James Elkins puts it, "Painting is an unspoken and largely uncognized dialogue, where paint speaks silently in masses and colors and the artist responds in moods" (Elkins, 2000, p. 5). Indeed, "as painters say, the paint seems to have a mind of its own – it 'wants' to do certain things, and it 'resists' the painter" (p. 121). In the same vein, painter and philosopher Nigel Wentworth maintains that, at its best, painting is a "vital interaction" that "allows the state of the painting at any one time to affect the direction the work takes, such that the painter can be led to do things that he had no prior intention of doing" (Wentworth, 2005, p. 51). Together these passages allude to three important features of the mutual give-and-take intrinsic to painting. First, they indicate that agentive 'others' have a *will* of their own and are therefore likely to respond and act in somewhat *unpredictable* ways. Vital interaction necessarily involves a potent element of surprise. Second, and connected to the previous, agentive interactants can never be completely brought under one's own *control*. The 'other' must be allowed to contribute to the dialogue if something new and vital is to be co-created. Third, painterly dialogue does not primarily take place on the level of analytical, reflective, and verbal thought. Rather, it operates in large part on a *preconscious* or *unconscious bodily-affective level*.

Painter Tarja Pitkänen-Walter registers each of these three features aptly when she writes:

> In artistic work, the most significant and vitalizing moment is when the artwork itself 'takes over the reins' and presents its maker with

> something unexpected. The artist's job is to follow that which has been "given" and to make subtle visual suggestions that support this exciting disclosure – all in the hope that that which has been revealed doesn't escape but instead, through one's choices, grows in strength. The most essential factor in creating a work of art is the appearance, nurturance, and pursuit of this "unknown". For the "unknown" brings with it a feeling of aliveness and vitality.
>
> (Saarinen, 2012b, p. 272, my translation)

Pitkänen-Walter goes on to observe that paintings do not typically remain at a rational and controllable distance from either their makers or their viewers. Rather, they "touch us" on the bodily, sensorial level much faster than on the cognitive one (p. 275). Thus, in what she calls an 'attitude of unknowing', the painter willingly relinquishes analytical discursive thinking in favor of a more associative, bodily-sensory, and non-verbal interaction.

To reiterate, we learn these basic experiential facts about creative reciprocity through recurrent exchanges with our nurturing environments. The key conditions of this early maturational process can be spelled out briefly as follows. In general, caregivers do not respond to their baby's experience in rigidly fixed patterns, nor do they reflect it back identically vis-à-vis the baby's perceptible behaviors. Rather, they recast the experience in variegated ways, typically cross-modally. This variation in affirmative responding not only supports the baby's emerging creative abilities but also intensifies the absorbing and exciting nature of the exchange itself. In these situations, the baby becomes highly alert to the caregiver's shifting expressions, vocalizations, kinetic and tactile responses, and so on. All the while, the baby begins to grasp that the caregiving environment is not under his magical control. Indeed, through sensitively enforced disillusionment, the baby comes to realize that his ability to mold the world according to his own needs and desires has its limits. In sum, early creative interaction is a dynamic and reciprocal affair, and, as such, proceeds in ways that cannot be entirely foreseen or controlled.

As suggested, these experiential elements of early interaction undergird the dialogical feel of mature artistic creation. With the vitalistic fantasy in force, the painting is expected to come to life and develop a will of its own. The painter also intuits that, if something novel and meaningful is to be created, she must surrender some of her own intentionality and permit the painting-as-other to contribute to the dialogue. Once the painting is perceived as an agentive collaborator rather than an object of unidirectional control, the painter will also become acutely aware of its changing qualities, and of what it has to 'say' or to 'suggest'. And, just as the baby seeks the thrill of his caregiver's shifting affirmative reactions, the painter hopes the painting will respond to her gestures in surprising, resonant, and vitalizing ways. She may even feel an urge to give in to the painting's will, and to thus let it 'carry' the creative process onward. At bottom, then, paintings spring to life through an open-ended give-and-take that is partially driven by archaic vitalistic fantasy.

The darker side of this fantasy is the possibility that the work will not come to life at all. Painter Richard Diebenkorn touches on this fear when he describes the beginning stages of each painting as follows: "What I do is face the blank canvas, which is terrifying. Finally, I put a few arbitrary marks on it that start me on some sort of dialogue. I need a dialogue to get going" (Gruen, 1991, p. 63). From a developmental point of view, the anxiety of facing a blank canvas can be seen to derive from a primal fear of not having one's strivings for vital contact satisfied. We need only view video clips (available online) from Edward Tronick's "still-face" experiments to apprehend the intensely negative feelings induced by unresponsive caregiving (see also Adamson & Frick, 2003; Tronick, 2003). In Tronick's set-up, the mother and child are initially engaged in playful and mutually responsive interaction. They coordinate their feelings and intentions together, face to face. Then the mother is asked to stop attending to her baby: she turns her head away for a second, and when she returns to face the baby, her expression is completely blank and unresponsive. The baby picks up on this immediately and does everything in its power to resume the prior state of vital connection, but to no avail. Eventually, the baby becomes extremely distressed and begins to cry. In a similar way, the painter must face a blank and unresponsive canvas with which she wishes to get a vital dialogue going. She needs the canvas to come to life, but at a deep level may fear that this will not happen. To overcome the initial trepidation, the painter must rely on the confidence and trust that she has built up through earlier successful creative interactions. However, even when the painting does come to life, there is still the possibility that it will become unresponsive or 'die' due to one's careless actions or misguided choices. Thus, as painter Leon Kossoff tells us, much artistic work inevitably consists in "discarding images that are dead" (Gayford, 2018, p. 136).

To sum up, I have maintained that the vitalistic fantasy contributing to the (potential) aliveness of paintings is rooted in and partially reenacts the creative dynamics of infant–caregiver interaction. Moreover, I have specified mutual responsiveness, relative unpredictability and uncontrollability, and the anticipation of affirmative form-giving as key elements of this dialogical give-and-take. I next turn to the third and final set of factors that makes paintings-in-progress liable to be experienced in a vitalistic way, namely, the material and metamorphic characteristics of paintings themselves.

The vital potential of paint and the metamorphosis of paintings

As specified in Chapter 2, different affective resources have different functions and properties, and therefore induce different forms of affective engagement and enhancement. Applying this notion to the arts, it is evident that musical sounds, written words, human bodies, paints on canvas, etc. each have dissimilar 'feels' to them. Simply put, each artistic medium has its unique sensory properties and potentialities, and hence affords distinct forms of creative manipulation and affective interaction. That being so, we may ask: What is it about paintings that sets them apart from other affective resources and simultaneously contributes to their special vitalistic appearance? In the following, I identify and discuss two factors. First, I investigate how paint, as a specific kind of material, looks and behaves. Second, I examine how paintings, as concrete objects made with paints, change and develop during the creative process. Throughout, I discuss how these material and metamorphic factors enable the special sense of aliveness that painters hold in such high value.

So, let us begin with paint itself. Graw seems to suggest that (traditional) oil paints have an intrinsic vitality of their own. She writes: "Pigments are harvested from nature and thus come with an *immanent aspect* of life and self-agency" (2018, p. 23, my italics). While this is an interesting observation, I find it somewhat mystifying. The link between ready-to-use oil paints and their origins in nature seems to me so tenuous that it can hardly account for the suggested vitalistic potential of paint. Besides, many pigments are gathered from minerals and other inorganic substances, which makes their connection to life and self-agency even more questionable. As it stands, I do not think Graw's suggestion can take us very far in explaining how paint enables paintings to come to life. Therefore, instead of dwelling on where paints come from, I propose we shift the spotlight to their characteristic 'look', 'feel', and 'behavior'.

One of the most striking features of paints is their capacity to form tissue-like layers and textures. Elkins, too, notes that paint can mimic living tissue by dint of its waxy, pliant, glossy, and smooth qualities (2000, p. 139). To add to this, he calls attention to the affinities between paints and various liquid elements involved in producing and balancing much organic life: "Liquids are life, and so it is particularly important that oil painting takes place between solid and liquid, in the realm of the viscous, the gluey, the phlegmatic" (pp. 166–167). Overall, in Elkins' view, the "substance that artists move around . . . has to come to life, or mimic life by shining, gleaming, catching the eye and ultimately living on its own" (p. 143). If and when painters adopt a similar attitude, they may relate to their paints as *dormant* materials, as if they were waiting in an intermediate state to be roused to life. Elkins also hints at this incipient state of possibility when he writes: "When the object is to make something living, it helps to begin with *half-living* ingredients" (pp. 140, my italics).

This kind of vitality of paint is considerably different from the type proposed by Graw. Although the vitality in question also involves inherent potentiality (which is there, at least, for painters), this potentiality is constituted by the *tangible material qualities* of the paints themselves rather than – and regardless of – their origins in the natural environment. In sum, the pliant materiality of paint can contribute to the organic feel of paintings in various ways, from forming tissue-like layers and textures to oozing and dripping like blood, phlegm, and other bodily fluids. Next, I want to elaborate on one such vitalistic effect, namely, the *skin-like* appearance of paint.

The membranous, epidermic character of paints and paintings has been discussed in particularly vivid fashion by psychoanalytical art critic Peter Fuller (1980, pp. 177–180, 207–213). In his extensive analysis of Robert Natkin's painting *Reveries of a Lapsed Narcissist*, Fuller reflects: "If you try to find words for what you see . . . you are most likely to pick on the word *skin*" (p. 177). To expand on this key impression, he describes the painting as "literally fleshy" and "undeniably saturated with a vibrant sensuality" (pp. 177–178). Indeed, from these vitalistic observations onward, Fuller's account takes on an explicitly carnal tone. He avows that the painting "is *attractive* almost in the sexual sense" and relates how the "eyes caress and explore it horizontally and vertically almost like hands moving across another's body in the fore-play to love-making" (p. 178). Eventually, one's vision is "seduced" and "compelled" to "penetrate deeper and deeper *inside* the painting", and once "the surface draws you *in*", the skin of paint is "reformed but this time *around you* so that you, originally an exterior observer, feel yourself to be literally and precariously suspended within a wholly illusory space" (pp. 178–179). Fuller adds that, personally, this sensation was not entirely positive, as it also elicited a foreboding sense of unease, anxiety, and terror (p. 208). Quite clearly, Fuller's description echoes the familiar trope of the painting as a female body and as an object of male desire. As art historian Rosemary Betterton bluntly comments, Fuller's aesthetic response closely and self-consciously "simulates the male sexual act: attraction, foreplay, penetration and, finally, release" (Betterton, 1996, p. 80). In short, his experiential account is problematically gendered to say the least.

However, when Fuller turns to theorize his experience in expressly Winnicottian terms, he unearths an important nugget of truth. As he sees it, the "formal mechanics" of Natkin's painting are "rooted in an immediate fashion in the *emotions and paradoxes of the 'potential space'*" (Fuller, 1980, p. 207, my italics). In this view, the appealing warmth and enveloping feel of the work are tied to "'very deep, very vague, and immensely generalized reminiscences,' which have to do with 'affection' and a 'sensuous co-existence' which at moments merges into a sense of fusion" (p. 207). There are three points worth highlighting here. First, what Fuller describes as deep and generalized reminiscences of sensuous coexistence, I have designated as vitalistic fantasy. The skin-like and flesh-like quality of paint evokes and supports this fantasy, and hence enhances the living feel of the painting. Second, the vitalistic fantasy, like creative interaction itself, plays out in the potential space, and thus involves unavoidable tensions between separateness and union, distance and proximity, and inner and outer. In line with this premise, Fuller notes that his unease at fusing with the painting owed to a primitive anxiety over losing himself completely or, in Winnicott's terms, of losing his basic sense of 'going on being' (p. 207). Third, as Betterton also points out, these particular aspects of Fuller's experience are essentially non-gendered, and therefore do not match particularly well with his strongly gendered description of responding to Natkin's painting. By mapping "an explicitly gendered, sexual reading of the painting on to a psychoanalytical explanation which deals with pre-Oedipal, non-gendered, experience", Fuller arguably makes a bit of a misstep (Betterton, 1996, p. 81).

On the whole, I believe that focusing on the Winnicottian aspects of Fuller's account gives us relevant insight not only into how an audience might feel in front of potentially vitalistic works but also into how *painters* may experience the skin-like and flesh-like qualities of their paints and paintings. These vitalistic effects may perhaps be even stronger for painters than for viewers, as painters interact with them in a concrete, hands-on, and highly invested manner. In sum, when the vitalistic fantasy is in effect, the painterly exchange may involve 'deep reminiscences of a sensuous co-existence' involving the other's skin, flesh, and body, and of accompanying feelings of warmth, envelopment, and being held. This, in turn, will boost the overall sense of the aliveness of the painting.

Before moving on, I want to say a few more words about the overall significance of paints for painters, for this too ties in with their vitalistic potential. As I have suggested, working with a specific medium can become deeply *entrenched* into the artist's overall sense of being (see Chapter 2). When this happens, the chosen medium may develop into an irreplaceable scaffold for highly valued ways of feeling, thinking, and making sense of the world. From this point of view, it is not surprising that many painters forge an exceptionally tight bond with the material of paint itself. Elkins describes this state of affairs as follows:

> To a nonpainter, oil paint is uninteresting and fairly unpleasant. To a painter, it is the *life's blood*: a substance so utterly entrancing, infuriating, and ravishingly beautiful that it makes it worthwhile to go back into the studio every morning, year after year, for an entire lifetime. As the decades go by, a painter's life becomes *a life lived with oil paint*, a story told in the thicknesses of oil.
>
> (2000, p. 5, my italics)

This is miles apart from a merely instrumental application of paint to achieve artistic ends. The painter's experiential life becomes inseparably entwined with the 'life' of her paints – she practically learns to feel and think through them.

When this kind of relationship is established, I believe that painters also become more inclined to experience their paints as organic matter. To put it rather simply, the more the artist and her paints share a life in the potential space, the more probable the extensive blending of subjective and objective, animate and inanimate, realities. Again, Elkins refers to this kind of experience when he writes: "Artists know the feeling that others can only weakly imagine, of being so close to their work that they cannot distinguish themselves from it" (2000, pp. 165–166). In this situation, "there is no clear difference between the artist and the half-formed work. Neither is in control, neither clearly 'makes' the other" (p. 166). I will discuss the details of such boundary dissolution in the next chapter. What is important for now is that, given the intimate bond between self and painting in such states, it is to be expected that any occurrent feeling of aliveness will permeate through the *entire* painter–painting dyad. When there is 'no clear difference between the artist and the half-formed work', there is also no longer such a sharp distinction between what is animate and what is not. As Elkins sums it up, "all that is known with certainty is the flow of fluids, back and forth from the tubes to the palette, from the brush to the canvas" (p. 166).

Lastly, I want to discuss the *metamorphic* factors that contribute to the felt aliveness of paintings. To clarify what metamorphosis means in this context, let us take a brief look at the general nature of organic life. Although there is no consensus over the properties – or combinations of properties – that are distinctive of life, there is agreement that these include some of the following. Living things change, grow, and develop; move and respond to stimuli; metabolize, reproduce, and die; and have complexly organized functional structures, heritable variability, and evolving lineages (Weber, 2018). Most or all of these characteristics are found together in animate matter, although some of them may appear selectively in inanimate matter as well.

Drawing from this, we might say that the outstanding vital features of paintings are 'responsiveness to stimuli' and 'change, development, and growth'. Of course, paintings cannot exhibit these qualities in any proper, intrinsic manner; they are merely attributed to inorganic matter through their makers' *experience*. Bearing this in mind, I suggest that the specified properties constitute the experienced metamorphic behavior of paintings. This means that, from the artist's point of view, paintings undergo *marked transformations*, both slowly and suddenly, and they do so by *responding* to the artist's own creative actions. Viewed in this light, painting may truly be called "the art of metamorphosis" (Elkins, 2000, p. 119).

The painter's main task is thus to manage the metamorphosis of her paintings. Elkins outlines two general approaches to this undertaking (2000, p. 121). On the one hand, painters have attempted to discipline and control their paints through conventionally learned practices and knowledge-based rules. In this approach, the transformation of paintings is typically brought about gradually and systematically, and by way of detailed plans and fixed methods. The painter might begin with preliminary drawings and studies to develop a clear course of action, move on to sketches and underpaintings on canvas, then proceed to apply painted layers and glazes, and finally finish the work with a coat of varnish. Elkins identifies the majority of pre-modern painters, the academicians of the eighteenth century, and most technically minded artists as exemplars of this methodic approach to painterly expertise and execution. On the other end of the spectrum, painters oversee the transformation of their paintings by allowing the paints to behave more freely, so that painting becomes a collaborative dialogue between the artist's gestures and the unpredictable tendencies of the paint itself. For these painters, "unexpected and inexplicable metamorphoses are the stock in trade of everyday work" (p. 146). In this group Elkins places the Expressionists, Neo-Expressionists, and the majority of contemporary painters. He also seems to find the latter approach more commendable, as indicated by the following observation: "No one knows what paint does, and when an artist is fooled into thinking paint can be entirely understood, then the studio becomes an annoying tedium where paint has to be pushed into place to make images" (p. 146).

It is reasonable to assume that painters working within a less rule-based and less rigidly methodical framework will tend to experience the development of their paintings more vitalistically. In other words, when control is loosened and paints are given relatively free rein, painters are more likely to experience their works as organic, agentive beings that 'have a say' in the creative process. From this experiential point of view, it makes perfect sense to speak of works as being 'nourished', 'kept alive', and 'grown' (Elkins, 2000, p. 144). Elkins has even suggested, somewhat fancifully, that paintings may be perceived as having *digestive* metabolic qualities. Seeing as the basic function of digestion is to decompose substances to extract essential components from them, elements undergoing digestion are by nature unsettled, as if in transition from one state to another, not quite this or that. Accordingly, Elkins observes that in paintings "[d]igestive areas are places where things almost are . . . they hold everything in suspension, letting the forms draw themselves almost into clarity" (p. 138). More specifically, "digestion happens in the warm darks", namely, in "passages of incipient shapes, of colors about to come into existence, and other colors fading away" (p. 139). Impressions of such intermediate states can become fixed features of particular areas of the finished painting and may therefore convey a sense of digestion not only to its maker but to its viewers, as well.

Finally, lingering above the transformation of paintings is the possibility of death. As Elkins observes, "any change is risky, and as painters know, even tried and true methods can go wrong" (2000, p. 141). However, risks must be taken if the painting is to be vital. It is "not enough to bring life to the inert pigments: the painter also has to toy with death, to bring the paint close to the point of no return in order to make it more convincing in the end" (p. 143). Metamorphosis may turn out to be fatal, and it is the painter's lot to manage this inherently precarious life-and-death endeavor. In keeping with this spirit of things, I will wrap up the chapter on a weighty existential note.

Existential vitality

Graw ends her discussion of the vitality of paintings with an incisive observation:

> Just as we are ceaselessly encouraged to become the agents of our own transformation, we certainly tend to treat art – and painting in particular – like a knowing and thinking agent *capable of effecting change*.
>
> (2018, p. 58, my italics)

On the one hand, this suggests that paintings can be projected as agents that make changes to themselves or, even more radically, as agents that have the power to bring themselves into existence. On the other hand, it implies that paintings are agents capable of effecting changes in *us* – their viewers and their makers. Indeed, I wish to emphasize that vital painterly interaction can have a great transformative impact on the person creating the painting. When paintings come alive and begin to metamorphose into beings of their own, their makers typically live and change alongside with them.

This transformative effect of paintings can be aptly illuminated by psychoanalyst Christopher Bollas's aesthetic theorization. Building on

Winnicott's thinking, Bollas (2018) designates as *transformational objects* those objects that have the power to induce significant changes in our experiential lives. The first and arguably most important in a long line of such objects is 'the caregiver'. To put it broadly, Bollas maintains that the baby's earliest experience of the caregiver is of a *process* that satisfies his needs and, accordingly, transforms his self-experience. That being so, the caregiver is not yet disclosed to the baby as an object as such but rather as a "recurrent experience of being". Early dyadic interaction therefore involves a "kind of existential, as opposed to representational, knowing" (pp. 89–90). Gradually, the baby comes to find and create objects apart from his caregivers that serve similar self-transformative functions – the primary example being transitional objects such as rags or soft toys (see Chapter 3). Later in life, transformational objects are sought more widely in the worlds of art, religion, ideology, and so on. At bottom, then, Bollas suggests that we are developmentally 'programmed' and existentially driven to pursue interactions with self-transforming and self-enhancing objects.

Importantly, in his discussion of transformational objects, Bollas discerns a close connection between early caregiving and later *aesthetic* experience:

> The mother's idiom of care and the infant's experience of the handling is one of the first if not the earliest human aesthetic. The uncanny pleasure of being held by a poem, a composition, a painting, or for that matter, any object, rests on these moments when the infant's internal world is partly given form by the mother since he cannot shape them or link them together without her coverage. The transformational object seems to promise the beseeching subject an experience where self-fragmentations will be integrated through a processing form.
>
> (Bollas, 1987, pp. 32–33)

By making art, we create 'processing forms' for ourselves and bring about the self-transformative experiences we so persistently desire. To put this in vitalistic, painterly terms, painting can provide us with the feeling of being in the presence of, and interacting with, a vital 'other' that holds us and makes us feel more alive, connected, and integrated.

I want to conclude by highlighting the fact that, according to Bollas, creative aesthetic experience involves an affectively constituted "existential recollection" (1987, p. 32). As he sums it up, "to seek the transformational object is really to recollect an early object experience, to remember not cognitively, but *existentially through intense affective experience*, a relationship that was identified with cumulative transformational experiences of the self" (2018, p. 91, my italics). This observation ties in directly with my view of painting as a means of dealing with the core existential concerns of life – that is, with concerns that fundamentally and perpetually bear upon our overall self–world relations. I have argued that these concerns are established in conjunction with the emergence of the potential space and, for that reason, are weaved into our being on a primal, preverbal, and bodily-affective level. Moreover, I have identified as one such fundamental concern the need to achieve a sense of vitality, or of feeling fully alive. And this is where the vitalistic potential of painting comes to play such a weighty existential role. By painting, the painter creates for herself a transformative affective scaffold: an object/process capable of satisfying her existential yearning for change and self-vitalization. Thus, painters do not bring their paintings to life only to enliven and advance the creative process but also so that they *themselves* can feel alive. Painting is therefore a special, existentially momentous relationship that scaffolds feelings that might be difficult for the painter to attain anywhere else.

Concluding remarks

In this chapter, I have discussed the special sense in which paintings-in-progress are experienced by their makers as organic and agentive beings. This is neither a delusion of aliveness nor, of course, does it imply a relationship with an actual living thing. Instead, it is a unique feeling supported by animistic myths and tropes; by unconscious fantasies, expectations, and relational dynamics; by the vitalistic material potentiality and metamorphic features of paints and paintings themselves; and, finally, by the artist's permissive approach to the unpredictable behavior of paints. The more weight each factor carries in the creative process, the more likely the painting is to be experienced as a living presence and interlocutor. To be sure, this is not a uniform affective state. Painters' feelings of their paintings' aliveness may be fleeting or prolonged, intense or mild, one-off or repeated, and may occur in various ways and forms – for instance, as a sense of dealing with something 'merely' organic or of engaging actively with something that possesses a will and power of its own. Finally, I have argued that the aliveness of one's paintings also enables *oneself* to feel more alive and connected. In this manner, the given feelings satisfy the core existential striving for vitalizing, meaningful, and enriching contacts with the surrounding world. For that reason, vitalistic feelings are deemed by many artists to be highly valuable and desirable.

Chapter 5

Oceanic feeling

The existential concern of demarcating and relating between self and not-self can affect the experience of painting in numerous ways. Perhaps its most striking manifestation is the blurring of boundaries between the painter and the painting – an occurrence that can in turn give rise to a wide range of feelings and perceptions. Consider, for example, the following observation by art critic Barry Schwabsky:

> When people paint – not for every kind of painting, but for more or less traditional painting that you do by hand with a brush or any kind of implement – there's a physical communication that goes from the surface of the support through the material that's on the end of the brush. Through the soft part of the brush, through the rigid part of the brush, to your hand, up your arm, and into your brain, and there is a loss of the sense of distinction between what's part of one's self and what's part of the objective world. I think that's where a certain 'mysticism' in painting comes from.
>
> (BOMB Magazine 118, 2012)

Here Schwabsky calls attention to the intermixing of the painter's body and the canvas: it is as if the bodily self and its extensions – hand, arm, and brush – merge together with the painting to produce a quasi-mystical feeling of union. Painter Stephen Newton describes experiencing something similar while working on one of his collage paintings:

> I began to paint at the top right hand corner . . . and was moving downwards when the vertical canvas seemed to slide down to a horizontal

> position. Suddenly and inexplicably, I found myself at the centre of an endless grey sea, with its surface covered as far as the eye could see with floating fragments or flotsam of canvas collage, scraps of line, painted and glued canvas, all rising and falling around my person half submerged at the centre of its infinity. I was not in any way fearful of drowning, being overwhelmed or lost; rather the experience was to be expected and welcomed and, at that time, didn't take me by surprise. When I was once again deposited on dry land, the painting had been completed.
>
> (Newton, 2008, p. 50)

Like Schwabsky, Newton describes a sense of bodily commingling with the painting, of somehow being submerged *in* the painting. This, he adds, amounts to a "peculiar sensation of envelopment . . . [in which] the whole womb of the painting draws you into itself in a total engulfment" (2008, p. 47). Moreover, Newton hints at a special mode of *perceiving* within the space of the painting: a way of seeing in which the material elements of the collage float, rise, and fall, fluidly and endlessly, as if on the waves of an ocean. Curiously, this state appears to have advanced the completion of his work.

Philosopher and painter Michael Krausz in turn recounts a life-changing experience amidst a series of large abstract canvases painted by a friend:

> I suddenly experienced myself in the space of the work instead of looking at it. More than that: I experienced an "interpenetration" of my self and the space of the painting. In that space, I suddenly became much more highly visually sensitive – to spatial relations, coloration and more.
>
> (Krausz, 2009, p. 191)

Krausz, like Newton, highlights how merging with the painting engendered an alternate and exceptionally sensitive way of seeing. Moreover, this episode implanted in Krausz an "inner necessity" to paint (p. 191). Crucially, he confirms that such 'interpenetrative' states continue to inform his ongoing artistic experience and practice.

At first view, the reported experiences might strike us as somewhat extraordinary – as aberrations from the normal processes of making art. However, a closer look at writings on aesthetics and artistic creativity suggests that feelings of dissolution and fusion are not all that rare while painting (see, e.g., Ehrenzweig, 1967; Hagman, 2005; Maclagan, 2001; Milner, 1957; Nelson & Rawlings, 2007; Newton, 2001; Rose, 1980; Saarinen, 2014b; Spitz, 1985; Townsend, 2019; Werman, 1986). As already suggested in relation to the *concreteness* of affective resources (Chapter 2), the separateness of paintings becomes a rather more flexible matter when considered from the artist's first-person point of view. This stands in stark contrast to the third-person perspective that inevitably discloses paintings as clearly distinct objects.

Unsurprisingly, a wide variety of terms and tropes have been put forward to describe these intriguing affective states. As Krausz points out,

> characterizations of nondualistic experiences might deploy such metaphors as "interpenetration" of subject and object, or "fusion" of artist and work, or "overcoming", or "dissolving", or "transcending" such binary opposites as subjective and objective reality. All these idioms suggest that, under particular circumstances, sharp distinctions between such binary terms as self and other, or subject and object, are undone.
>
> (2009, p. 194)

Krausz also notes that, depending on one's preferred theoretical orientation, these states have been designated as "nirvanic, epiphanic, numinous, religious, flow, ecstatic, or oceanic" (p. 194). Because the term 'oceanic' has become relatively well established in psychoanalytical (aesthetic) theorization, I adopt it as my term of choice in this chapter.

In what follows, I examine dissolution and fusion experiences in painting via three key questions. First, what does the oceanic feeling *feel* like? Second, what kinds of factors give rise to the feeling and contribute to its experiential unfolding? And finally, why do some painters consider the oceanic state highly valuable to their creative work? To address these questions, I first provide a historical synopsis of 'oceanic feeling' in psychoanalytical theorization. I then elaborate on the experiential features, generative mechanisms, and potential value of the feeling vis-à-vis ongoing theoretical debate on the topic. The purpose of this preliminary overview is to clarify my use of the concept and to set up the second part of the chapter, in which I analyze the oceanic feeling in the specific context of painterly creativity.

What is the oceanic feeling?

The concept of the oceanic feeling emerged into psychoanalytical theorization from the correspondence between Sigmund Freud and Romain Rolland in the first half of the twentieth century (for an in-depth study, see Parsons, 1999; see also Saarinen, 2012a, 2014b; Maharaj, 2017). Besides being a Nobel Prize-winning novelist and social critic, Rolland was a professed mystic who had in his youth experienced several rapturous feelings of union, limitlessness, and eternity. As he matured, these transient mystical episodes consolidated into a more permanent way of being or, as one might argue, into an overall existential orientation (Saarinen, 2014b). In Rolland's terms, at the core of this developmental achievement was "the simple and direct fact of *the feeling of the 'eternal'* (which, can very well not be eternal, but simply without perceptible limits, and like oceanic, as it were)" (quoted in Parsons, 1999, p. 173, emphasis in original). Rolland (1930) maintained that the oceanic feeling not only provided a valuable sense of vitality and strong moral fiber but also revealed the mind's inherent connectedness to a supra-individual and limitless metaphysical substance. Seeking to discuss the psychological fundaments of his view, Rolland turned to Freud for a psychoanalytic interpretation of the matter.

Freud, who claimed never to have experienced anything of the kind, was somewhat perplexed by Rolland's request. He nonetheless presented a tentative analysis of the oceanic feeling in the first chapter of *Civilization and Its Discontents* (1930). After rephrasing its ideational contents as that of "limitlessness and of a bond with the universe" and of "an indissoluble bond, of being one with the external world as a whole", Freud explained the feeling in terms of individual development (p. 65). He reasoned that a primary "all-embracing feeling" of infant–mother unity could endure "side by side with the narrower and more sharply demarcated ego feeling of maturity" (p. 68). Simply put, Freud found the roots of the oceanic feeling in the benign preservation of primary narcissism. As such, it was a remnant of the past that could affect the present but was nonetheless bereft of any adaptive value for day-to-day living. In the end, Freud and Rolland failed to find agreement over the basic nature and value of the oceanic feeling.

In the immediate period following Freud's analysis, the term was often used in psychoanalytic writing as a euphemism for unitive mystical experiences that were deemed defensive, infantile, and pathological – thus divorcing it even further from Rolland's original, commendatory stance. In the late 1950s and early 1960s, however, more charitable psychoanalytical views towards mysticism began to emerge. At the same time, the oceanic feeling became increasingly applied to phenomena beyond the religio-mystical domain, most notably to aesthetic experience and artistic creativity (see, e.g., Ehrenzweig, 1953, 1967; Milner, 1957; Stokes, 1955). As its use proliferated, the concept gained in theoretical nuance and sparked further debate about the feeling's experiential features, generating mechanisms, and potential value. I address each of these issues in turn next.

Feeling oceanic

The predominant view of the affective essence of the oceanic feeling is voiced by psychoanalyst Joel Kovel, who characterizes it as the "sense of being one with the universe and of dissolving the boundaries of the ego" (1990, p. 71). Put simply, *fusion* and *self-boundary dissolution* are commonly regarded as the core experiential features of the oceanic feeling: the two appear together systematically and are practically inseparable. Behind this façade of general consensus, however, things get a little bit more complicated. For example, scholar of religion Robert K. C. Forman (1998) has proposed that the oceanic feeling is merely a *precursor* to potential feelings of oneness. He defines the oceanic feeling as a dualist state of self-expansion in which one's awareness is field-like and unbounded, and only gradually broadens beyond the limits of the body. This state can then evolve into a unitive mystical episode in which the unbounded self is experienced to permeate and merge with things in the world. Interestingly, studies on synesthesia and sexual ecstasy (Nielsen, Kruger, Hartmann, Passie, Fehr, & Zedler, 2013) and hallucinogen-induced altered states of consciousness (Vollenweider, Gamma, & Vollenweider-Scherpenhuyzen, 1999; Vollenweider, 2001) have also designated as 'oceanic boundlessness' the peculiar sense of dissolving boundaries. This research likewise suggests that dissolution can begin with a mere loosening of ego-boundaries, which may (or may not) then culminate in a feeling of merger with the universe (and hence, a full-blown mystical state of oneness) (Vollenweider et al., 1999).

On the other hand, even when the oceanic feeling has been identified primarily as a feeling of oneness, opinions have diverged as to *what* the subject can feel at one with. While some authors have claimed that the oceanic state is a feeling of oneness with the universe exclusively (see, e.g., Goldie, 2008), many others have suggested that it can take on more specific objects as well, including deities (Mills, 1999), music (Kohut, 2011), meditational objects (Epstein, 1990), parts of nature (Koestler, 1954), and, of course, works of art (Stokes, 1978; Milner, 1957, 1987; Ehrenzweig, 1967; Wolson, 1995; Newton, 2001). If we take the latter, more inclusive approach, most if not all feelings of fusion are effectively classifiable as oceanic. Novelist Arthur Koestler captures this broad stance nicely: "That higher entity, of which the self feels a part, to which it surrenders its identity, may be nature, God, the anima mundi, the magic of form, or the ocean of sound" (2009, p. 258).

Deciding which experiential features are constitutive of the oceanic feeling 'proper' is, in the final analysis, a somewhat arbitrary matter. It is, after all, a fluid construct that is tied to shifting theoretical purposes and commitments. One can, for example, take a strictly minimalist position – as I have done elsewhere in maintaining that the feeling of self-boundary dissolution is not only a necessary condition for oceanic feeling but also a *sufficient* one in its own right (Saarinen, 2014b). On that account, any feeling of fusion, merger, or oneness with a given object (including artworks) is a secondary and contingent upshot of the oceanic feeling rather than its constitutive and distinctive property. Having said that, in the present study I will use 'oceanic feeling' in a much more permissive sense – that is, to denote a broader class of feeling that frequently includes fusion with individual objects as well.

I adopt this approach with several specifications in mind. First, I use the terms 'fusion' and 'self-dissolution' as bywords for various *closely related feelings*. I take 'fusion' to encompass a family of feelings including engulfment, intermingling, interpenetration, oneness, merger, union, and the like, whereas 'dissolution' is meant to accommodate feelings of disintegration, blurring, expansion, boundlessness, limitlessness, and so on. To be clear, I do not mean to imply that all feelings grouped under one or the other – that is, under 'fusion' or 'dissolution' – are experientially identical to each other. The purpose is instead to corral two families of interconnected feelings into sufficiently manageable terminological confines.

Second, it should be noted that the *experiential relations* between fusion and dissolution can be quite complex. Suffice it to say that feelings of dissolution do not necessarily lead to feelings of fusion, either with particular things or the world in general, nor is it entirely clear that feelings of fusion must presuppose any conscious experience of boundary dissolution. From this point of view, oceanic feelings can be experienced as either (1) devoid of any ascribable intentional object or (2) as involving an intentional object – be it specific or non-specific, real or imagined. In the former case, self-boundary dissolution dispenses with specific intentional relatedness to one's surroundings but does not amount to a feeling of oneness or fusion with any particular objects. For lack of a better term, we may call such cases diffuse or pure oceanic feelings. In the second case, the experience of self-boundary dissolution is accompanied by intentional directedness towards some object or another. Perhaps all cases of self-boundary dissolution that *do* involve an intentional object necessarily entail a feeling of fusion or oneness with that object (seeing as the boundaries between the self and the object are experienced as dissipated). Thus, the experience of self-boundary dissolution in relation to a painting will entail a feeling of fusion with that painting.

Third, feelings of dissolution and fusion *come in degrees*: from minor commixtures of self and world to all-embracing states of boundlessness and union. Typically, states that have been designated as 'oceanic' entail quite *noticeable* degrees of dissolution and/or fusion; I also subscribe to this general view here. Finally, as suggested by Newton and Krausz, oceanic feelings tend to include notable changes in one's experience of *bodily* boundaries, in one's *perceptions* of objects and their boundaries, and also in one's overall *psychological* grasp of what is self and what is not-self. These three elements overlap and become experientially accentuated in different ways in different cases of oceanic feeling.

All in all, it would be an immense task to dissect the experiential structure of all variations of oceanic feeling, even within the limited context of painting. I will therefore highlight only some variants in the second part of the chapter, with a special emphasis on the *perceptual* features of creative oceanic states. But next, I discuss the possible sources and generating mechanisms of oceanic feeling.

Into the ocean deep

Following Freud, many psychoanalytically oriented theorists and researchers have explained the oceanic feeling in terms of *regression to an infantile developmental state*. The guiding premise in these accounts is that neonates inhabit a fundamental state of ego-undifferentiation and infant–mother unity (see also the discussion of Winnicott in Chapter 3). An affective, presymbolic memory of this state persists and can subsequently be revived in oceanic experience. For example, Margaret Mahler, Fred Pine, and Anni Bergman famously identified "normal symbiosis" as "that state of undifferentiation, of fusion with mother, in which 'I' is not yet differentiated from the 'not-I' and in which inside and outside are only gradually coming to be sensed as different" (1989, p. 44). Based on this, they surmised that the "dual unity within one common boundary . . . is perhaps what Freud and Romain Rolland discussed in their dialogue as the sense of boundlessness of the oceanic feeling" (p. 44).

Kevin Fauteux (1994) and Mortimer Ostow (2007) have followed a similar line of reasoning. Fauteux maintains that the adult oceanic experience regressively restores the symbiotic state, albeit imperfectly, and in doing so revives early feelings of tranquility, passivity, and unity. As he puts it, "symbiotic unity still seems the most incisive way to describe unitive oceanic experience and the archaic infant-maternal matrix it restores" (1994, p. 222). Ostow in turn reflects:

> If our thoughts about regression are correct, then the oceanic feeling may reproduce the feeling that the infant has lost when he begins to appreciate that he and his mother are two separate individuals. The mystic's yearning for union then expresses the wish to reunite with the mother into a symbiotic unit.
>
> (2007, p. 46)

Ostow emphasizes that the oceanic feeling does not gratify this wish in mere imagination; instead, it involves the genuine reactivation of "a complex of affects and dispositions that prevailed early in childhood" (p. 69).

To reiterate, these and other similar explanations hinge on the notion of primary infant–caregiver unity. In the past few decades, however, this premise has been increasingly questioned in both clinical psychoanalysis and empirical infant research. Much of the evidence suggests that there is no absolute phase of symbiosis or undifferentiation to which the individual can later return or regress (for discussions about this issue, see, e.g., Peterfreund, 1978; Eigen, 1983; Horner, 1985; Stern, 1985; Harrison, 1986; Lachmann & Beebe, 1989; Merkur, 1999; Rochat, 2003; Pine, 2004; Silverman, 2004; Reddy, 2008; Taipale, 2014). Indeed, neonates appear to be capable of a rudimentary form of non-reflexive self-awareness, engaging with their environments in ways that bear witness to their ability to distinguish themselves from others. In accordance with this view, some authors have suggested that the oceanic feeling is due to a regressive and/or wish-fulfilling *fantasy* rather than the re-evocation of a prior state (Harrison, 1986; Lachmann & Beebe, 1989). Irving B. Harrison, for example, has argued that there is "no basis for the assumption that the oceanic feeling exists in normal infants or children"; hence "the fact that some adults experience oceanic feelings does not imply that they represent the original psychic state of the neonate" (1986, p. 156, 157). He concludes that "nothing is returned to, in the extreme regression of the oceanic feeling, except in fantasy" (p. 156). On this view, the oceanic feeling is not a return to a prior state; however, it is still unmistakably regressive in its reversion to an infantile and hallucinatory form of wish fulfillment.

More recently, Joona Taipale (2014) has put forward an account that elegantly seeks to reconcile key elements from both primary unity theories and theories that advocate primary differentiation. He maintains that infantile experience consists of two co-constitutive aspects: pleasure-seeking fantasy and factual kinesthetic feel, perception, etc. Whereas moments of merger take place in the register of fantasy, moments of differentiation take place in the register of bodily fact. During the course of infantile experience, one or the other register can become dominant, leading to corresponding experiential shifts along the unity–differentiation continuum. Michael Eigen (1983) has similarly suggested that union and separateness occur together, with one or the other being more pronounced in any given situation. He introduces the term 'dual union' to "refer to the simultaneous presence of both distinction and union dimensions", this being a basic structure that characterizes the self on all of its developmental levels (p. 425). Accordingly, Eigen prefers to speak of soft, permeable, and changing boundaries that may shift towards the extremes of union or distinction.

I find the accounts proposed by Taipale and Eigen appealing because they avoid rigid either/or assumptions about the primary nature of infantile experience. As I previously suggested in my discussion of Winnicott's view of early unity (Chapter 3), it is arguable that the infant cannot yet *consistently* and *clearly* distinguish its caregiving objects from itself. We can thus hold on to the idea that a considerable part of early experiencing consists in feelings of undifferentiation or, perhaps more accurately, of notably fluid and wavering self–other boundaries. Importantly, this does not exclude the possibility of concurrent experiences of rudimentary self-differentiation and separateness.

This brings us back to the issue of regression. I find more appealing those accounts that either minimize its role in explaining oceanic feeling or dispense with the notion altogether (see Ehrenzweig, 1967; Werman, 1986; Storr, 1989; Kovel, 1990; Merkur, 1999; Loewald, 2000; Meissner, 2005). Even though many of these accounts continue to subscribe to some variant of neonatal unity/symbiosis, they opt to explain the oceanic feeling in terms of *present-day, fully developed psychological functioning*. As David Werman (1986) puts it,

> although the relative absence of boundaries in the infant may be the *prototype* for the oceanic experience and for states of consciousness where self-boundaries are blurred or disappear altogether, it is clear that these experiences are not simple regressions to an infantile level. The oceanic experience . . . is an *adult* phenomenon which in no significant manner can be duplicated by the infant.
>
> (p. 136, emphasis in original)

Kovel (1990) likewise maintains that an infantile prototype of the oceanic feeling exists and can consequently affect later experience. Even so, he asks: "Is there . . . nothing left over to the oceanic experience once its infantile roots have been laid bare?" (1990, p. 74) By way of response, Kovel postulates a critical difference between infant and adult oceanic experiencing, suggesting that "the infantile prototype of the oceanic experience must be in essence a moment of *falling asleep*, of *losing consciousness*", whereas "all religious oceanic moments are marked by an *awakening*, or a *gaining* of consciousness – not the discharge of tension" (p. 74, emphasis in original). Whether or not these blanket statements about infantile and religious oceanic experience are entirely correct – and I suspect they are not – the general point holds. That is,

> [the] infantile version of the oceanic experience is simply that – a *version*, or to use another term, an occasion. . . . Thus we need not assume that later versions of the oceanic experience are somehow produced by the memory of the first one.
>
> (p. 76, emphasis in original)

In sum, even if the adult oceanic feeling is in some respects influenced by ontogenetic factors, it exceeds the explanatory bounds of mere regressive-developmental dynamics.

A feasible way to circumvent the thorny issues of regression and primary differentiation/undifferentiation is to explain adult oceanic feeling in terms of two intertwined, developed *modes of mentation*. This type of approach is exemplified by psychiatrist and mysticism scholar Arthur Deikman (1971), who distinguishes between the “action” and “receptive” modes of consciousness. The former is oriented towards biological survival via active manipulation of the environment, and therefore “requires a clear sense of self-object difference” (p. 481). The receptive mode is in turn organized around the intake of the environment. Its key attributes include “diffuse attending, paralogical thought processes, decreased boundary perception, and the dominance of the sensory over the formal” (p. 481). Everyday experience consists in ongoing balancing between, and intermixing of, these two modes. However, Deikman points out that the action mode typically comes to dominate in adulthood and thus tends to be regarded as the ‘proper’ one, whereas the more unusual and intermittent receptive mode tends to be (wrongly) seen as regressive or pathological.

Based on this bimodal model of consciousness, Deikman argues that states of self-boundary dissolution and unity are produced by *de-automatization* – that is, by an “undoing of the automatic psychological structures that organize, limit, select, and interpret perceptual stimuli” (1971, p. 487; see also Deikman, 1966; Geels, 1982). In short, de-automatization loosens the hold on experience of the action mode of perception and, in doing so, allows the receptive mode to take over. Crucially, Deikman maintains that de-automatization is not a regressive return to childhood – even if the receptive mode originates and functions maximally in infancy (1966, p. 331; 1971, p. 481). As he puts it, “one might call the direction regressive in a developmental sense, but the actual experience is probably not within the psychological scope of any child” (1966, p. 331). Rather, “it is a de-automatization occurring in an adult mind, and the experience gains its richness from adult memories and functions now subject to a different mode of consciousness” (p. 331). To be clear, the ‘different’ mode of consciousness Deikman refers to here is the receptive mode, which is “a mature cognitive and perceptual state, one that is not ordinarily dominant, but is an option that has developed in richness and subtlety in parallel with the development of the action mode that is our customary state of consciousness" (1971, p. 487).

In strikingly similar fashion, art pedagogue and critic Anton Ehrenzweig (1967) has argued that the mind (or the ego) is essentially two-tiered by nature, divided into opposing levels of surface and depth mind. He maintains that these two levels incorporate distinct modes of attention and perception. Differentiated surface-level attention produces consciously controlled, narrowly focused, and distinctly articulated perception, whereas dedifferentiated depth-level attention produces unconscious, fluid, diffuse, and holistic perception. In other words, the surface mind tends to present things as clearly separate, whereas the depth mind tends towards loosening their boundaries, freely mixing and merging them together. At any given moment, attention oscillates between these extreme ends and thus incorporates various levels of perception simultaneously. Like Deikman, Ehrenzweig argues that the oceanic state "need not be due to a 'regression', to an infantile state, but could be the product of the extreme dedifferentiation in lower levels of the ego" (1967, p. 294). As the undifferentiated mode of perception disrupts differentiated conscious perception, it can remove "the boundaries of individual existence and so produce a mystic oceanic feeling that is distinctively manic in quality" (p. 294).

Following Deikman and Ehrenzweig, I also maintain that an undifferentiated mode of mentation plays a key role in the emergence of adult oceanic feelings (Saarinen, 2012b). In simplified terms, the oceanic feeling occurs when this mode blends into or extensively displaces the more differentiated one. I will return to this notion later in this chapter, in the context of painting. But before that, I will conclude the first part of this chapter with an overview of the debate over the value of the oceanic feeling.

The question of value

As mentioned, a major point of contention between Rolland and Freud was the *value* of the oceanic feeling. Rolland maintained that the benefits of the feeling were multiple: it could deliver knowledge of immutable metaphysical truths; guide socio-ethical behavior; inspire creativity; constitute a non-dogmatic religious life; and vitalize one's entire being. Freud, on the contrary, expressly denied that the oceanic state was either a reliable source of knowledge or suitable for adaptation to the surrounding world.

He did, however, suggest that the restoration of all-encompassing primary narcissism could play a consolatory role by denying outside threats to the ego (1930, p. 72).

The thoughts about value expressed in the correspondence between Rolland and Freud have re-emerged in various forms in subsequent debates on the oceanic feeling (see Parsons, 1999). Attitudes towards its value can be broadly categorized into three groups: principally negative, principally positive, and neutral. Accounts in the negative group take a highly skeptical or straightforwardly rejective stance towards the possibility of positive value. This position tends to go hand in hand with viewing the oceanic feeling as a pathological form of psychological defense. Jeffrey M. Masson (1980), for instance, has claimed in his early writings that psychoanalysis can reveal the defensive and pathological nature of most, if not all, religio-mystical experience and behavior. Typical of, for example, asceticism is the defensive flight from a disconcerting (inner) reality. The inability to recognize or face such basic emotions as loss, sadness, and the yearning for contact leads to a detachment from healthy human relations – the only source of authentic happiness (1980, pp. 1–16). Thus, the "desire for union [in the oceanic feeling] is both an attempt to deny a deeper need for companionship, and a means of displaying totally-disguised annihilation fantasies" (p. 70). Harrison argues the same point: "The oceanic feeling as observed in adults is a symptom, incorporating a defensive maneuver, comparable to a delusion denying the fact of intense distress" (1986, p. 156). In sum, from this perspective the oceanic feeling is a negative denial of basic human need and a psychopathological retreat from an unsatisfying world.

On the other end of the spectrum, the oceanic feeling is considered to be highly valuable and hence commendable. Several authors have discussed the positive effects of the feeling on specific activities, most notably on artistic creativity (Ehrenzweig, 1967; Milner, 1987; Rooney, 2007; Newton, 2008; Krausz, 2009). Others have highlighted its benefits to social life and to living in general. David M. Levin (1988), for instance, views the feeling as grounds for subverting a metaphysics that promotes unjustifiably rigid subject–object distinctions. Ultimately, he sets his sights on comprehensive social reform:

> What I have in mind, then, is a movement which is not (so to speak) "completed" until the "oceanic" experience, the wisdom of

> interconnectedness and wholeness, has been brought back, brought into the present, and appropriately integrated into present living.
>
> (pp. 218–219)

This brings us to the third and final approach to value. Accounts in this group recognize that oceanic feelings can have various psychological functions, including goal-oriented, adaptive, defensive, destructive, and creative functions (see, e.g., Werman, 1986; Parsons, 1999; Goldie, 2008). As a consequence, these accounts are less likely to promulgate straightforwardly negative or positive evaluations of the feeling. I, too, endorse this type of view. That is to say, I believe that the value of the oceanic feeling can be highly variable. Consider philosopher André Comte-Sponville's remarks about the effects of his personal oceanic experiences:

> Though few and far between, these experiences have changed my daily life, making it a bit less heavy – and even, on good days, happier. They have lastingly transformed my relationship to the world, to other people, to myself, to art . . . to philosophy, to spirituality.
>
> (Comte-Sponville, 2008, p. 159)

It would be a stretch to argue that Comte-Sponville's oceanic experiences are world-weary or delusional. On the other hand, the feeling can also be symptomatic of psychopathology or open to manipulation by others with morally suspect motives. While generally valuing the feeling highly, Kovel recognizes "that the state of connectedness, or the oceanic consciousness that accompanies it, is not in itself a good thing", and cites the Nazi movement's exploitation of "oceanic release" as a notoriously malignant example (1990, p. 86).

Finally, it is worth emphasizing that the value of oceanic feeling is neither reducible to nor explained away by its generating mechanisms. As philosopher Peter Goldie observes, we can remain neutral about the origins of the oceanic feeling "whilst we are concerned with its ideational contents in mature adults, and whilst we are concerned with its value" (2008). To assess whether a given instance of the oceanic feeling is beneficial or detrimental, we might consider any number of factors, including its outcomes and contextual appropriateness. Fauteux (1995) suggests that a deciding factor is whether the feeling occurs in the service of the ego. For the oceanic state to be beneficent, one must "play with" the primary process it uncovers, "return to the world", and "act on" the experience (p. 81; see also Kris, 1952). Moreover, he claims that "the experience must be transient, not clung to, even though a regressive urge to remain may exist" (p. 160). Clinging to the feeling, Fauteux warns us, can lead to a sense of being overwhelmed and lost, or even to psychosis.

At this point, we can summarize the preparatory part of this chapter. For present purposes, I have committed myself to three basic premises. First, I define the oceanic feeling broadly as a feeling of self-boundary dissolution and/or fusion. What one fuses with can be an individual object or one's surroundings in general. Second, instead of explaining the feeling as a regression to infantile symbiosis or, for that matter, in primarily developmental terms to begin with, I examine its emergence within the framework of a mature, bimodally structured mind. Finally, I hold that, whatever its generating mechanisms, the feeling's value depends on its overall context and outcomes. With these theoretical settings in place, I will now analyze the oceanic feeling in the context of painterly creativity.

The oceanic feeling in painterly creativity

While painting, the artist inhabits an experiential space wherein sharply demarcated boundaries between subjective and objective, self and not-self, are liable to dissolve, intermix, and reform in various vivid ways. As Gilbert Rose puts it, in painting "subject, object, and interaction become interwoven in a dynamic system: a temporary sense of fusion is followed by reseparation, a dissolution of inner boundaries is followed by a redelineation" (1980, p. 13). Accordingly, he describes the essence of artistic creativity as "controlled play with the boundaries of reality" (p. 72), which alludes aptly to the core existential concern of self–other demarcation (see Chapter 3). From this point of view, it is not surprising that the boundaries of the self can become exceptionally fluid and permeable while painting, and that painters may experience, to varying degrees, oceanic feelings of dissolution and fusion with their works-in-progress. Although full-scale feelings of oneness with paintings are not completely unheard of, it is far more common for painters to experience their works simultaneously as parts of themselves *and* as parts of the material world, that is, without the two realms merging completely into one. It is this latter, more *moderate* type of oceanic feeling that I examine here.

To gain a better grasp of the matter, let us return to Krausz's and Newton's portrayals of their personal oceanic experiences. Krausz highlights the significance of the feeling for his own artistic work by citing philosopher Arthur Danto, who considers states of unity to be the "high moments of artistic work, those moments of pure creativity, when artist and work are not separated by a gap of any sort, but fuse in such a way that the work seems to bring itself into existence". Danto continues: "At such points – and any creative person lives for these – there is none of the struggle and externality that marks those phases of artistic labor in which inspiration fails and the work itself refuses to cooperate" (Krausz, 2009, p. 194; from Danto, 1972, pp. 110–111). Newton, too, asserts that the oceanic state "forms the very fulcrum" of the creative process (2008, p. 104), as only it can afford "the conditions for a complete breakdown of conscious functioning and a reformulation of psychic structure as the mind is externalised and reconstituted or embodied within the evolving artwork" (p. 93). These excerpts certainly point toward the benefits of the oceanic feeling for painting. But what, more specifically, could account for holding it in such high regard? In what ways can oceanic experience affect artistic creativity positively?

Krausz and Newton approach these questions with differing intuitions and assumptions. In fact, after quoting Danto approvingly, Krausz leads the discussion into a somewhat surprising direction. Whereas Danto (in the given passage) indicates that the state of fusion is *integral* to the ongoing artist–artwork interaction, Krausz suggests that, during its occurrence, the oceanic state actually *excludes* the possibility of creative activity. He writes:

> Indeed, for their duration, nondualistic experiences do inhibit creative activity. For the ability of emergent properties of a work to affect their creator depends upon a duality between creator and work. . . . Such duality is necessary for the creator to be 'carried by' or 'influenced by' the creator's work in progress.
>
> (Krausz, 2009, p. 196)

Simply put, in this view, the oceanic state puts the actual activity of creating art on hold. Krausz contends that this is necessarily so because the capacity to react to the developing features of the work presupposes a clear experiential distinction between painter and painting. During a state of fusion the painter could not, for example, apply paint to the canvas and then adjust any imbalance caused by these marks to the overall composition of the painting. This kind of action sequence would require a detached perspective from which the painting would again be disclosed as a distinct object of manipulation and evaluation.

If Krausz is right, the benefits of the oceanic feeling for painterly creativity are at best *indirect*, coming into effect only after the affective state runs its course and sufficient separateness is once again reinstated. Indeed, Krausz affirms that the "afterglow" of the experience can "inform" subsequent 'dualist' creative work (2009, p. 196). He also suggests that oceanic feelings can inspire creativity more generally, as elements of an artistically creative life or as parts of artistic projects that aim at creative self-transformation (p. 197). I certainly agree that oceanic feelings can affect one's painterly activities in various indirect, yet decisive and long-lasting, ways (Saarinen, 2014b). Intense episodes of dissolution and fusion can cause dramatic and permanent shifts in one's overall sense of reality. It is no surprise that such fundamental changes in how one finds oneself in the world can also reconfigure the motives, methods, and aims of one's artistic efforts. In this situation, the painter's art-making process is not so much affected by concurrent oceanic states as by an underlying existential orientation that has become partly established via prior episodes of oceanic feeling.

But what matters here is that, in Krausz's account, the oceanic feeling is somewhat disconnected from the hands-on activity of painting – from those decisive moments when brush meets canvas and the painting is worked towards its completion. This gives rise to a decisive question: is it really the case that oceanic experience categorically curtails all simultaneous creative activity? In this regard, Newton turns out to be at odds with Krausz. Case in point, Newton claims that his collage painting was successfully completed during an extended period of oceanic submergence (2008, p. 50) – thus echoing Danto's observation about the 'work seemingly bringing itself into existence' in a state of painter–painting unity. This possibility is also supported by visual artist Patricia Townsend (2019), who describes the feeling of unity with her own work of art as follows: "I did feel a sense of oneness with the developing work. However, in retrospect, it did not seem to me that I moved out of that state in order to make moment-to-moment decisions about . . . practical questions" (p. 56). The essential implication here is that fusion does not necessarily exclude attending to, acting on, or reacting to the object one is concurrently merged with.

To clarify this phenomenon by way of comparison, let us take a brief look at feelings of fusion between two persons. Consider the activity of partner dancing. During the dance, two bodies become coupled through coordinated interactions to produce a "dyadic bodily state" (Fuchs & De Jaegher, 2009, p. 472). Experientially, this amounts to a momentary blurring of the boundaries between the coupled subjects. However, a degree of awareness of relating to the other as an 'other' still remains. It's not as if one felt like he or she were dancing with oneself. Rather, it is only when both dancers are sufficiently sensitive and responsive to each other's movements that the dance can proceed smoothly. What's particularly relevant about this dyadic, coupled state is how the dancers *attend* to and *react* to the ongoing process. They perceive and process an abundance of changing stimuli to which they then simultaneously and appropriately respond. However, and this is critical, the dancers need not *consciously reflect* on the other's movements, nor do they need to *consciously deliberate* on how they should respond to them. In fact, excessive reflection on these matters would in all likelihood disrupt the flow of the dancing. This indicates that in states of fusion the capacity to act on and react to fused-with objects can indeed function effectively; these processes just tend to take place outside full reflective awareness and deliberation.

I believe that a similar mechanism applies to painting during oceanic states of merger. As suggested in Chapter 2, in the bidirectional activity of painting the developing work becomes part of a tightly coupled painter–painting feedback loop. Under these circumstances, the painting is experienced as both part of the self and as an 'other': a presence that responds to one's painterly gestures by shutting down certain possibilities while opening up others, and by resisting, suggesting, or even demanding further courses of action. The artist must thus remain attentive and responsive to these changing, cue-like features of the painting. As in the dancing, the oceanic state does not necessarily disrupt this type of painterly activity. Rather, it constitutes a special interactive state in which reflective deliberation over appropriate courses of action is significantly diminished. When one loses oneself in dance or in painting, the activity carries itself, as it were.

At this point the objection could be raised that, even if the oceanic state allows for attentive-responsive activity, it still inhibits *creative* activity. In other words, one might argue that there is some necessary condition of creative activity that the oceanic feeling effectively negates; most evidently, perhaps, the ability to *evaluate critically* one's developing work. Krausz makes this very point in claiming that "nonduality inhibits criticism and critical interaction between creator and work" (2009, p. 196). To be sure, I agree that critically analyzing and editing one's work is a crucial element in nearly all successful artistic creation. However, I suggest that evaluative assessment typically comes in two types. Whereas the aforementioned critical evaluation is carried out from the dualist position of detachment and distance, the second, absorbed type evaluates the 'rightness' or 'goodness' of the work while one is fully immersed in the activity of painting. This type of assessment is fast, intuitive, and mostly subconscious, and is just as important as disengaged contemplation for the overall creative cycle. Townsend touches on the same phenomenon when she describes her own evaluative activity and decision-making in a state of absorptive oneness as follows: "*at the same time*, I was making practical decisions. Indeed, I could only make appropriate decisions if I retained my close connection, or sense of 'oneness', with the work, as I needed to sense whether the changes I made brought it closer to, or further from, my inner experience" (2019, p. 56, emphasis in original). In short, I concur with Krausz that clearly detached critical observation is (by definition) incompatible with oceanic feeling. However, this is but one aspect of the creative process, and leaves plenty of room for the other type of evaluative responsiveness to operate in oceanic states of merger, as described by Newton and Townsend.

In sum, if we grant that painting is indeed possible during oceanic states and, moreover, want to argue that these states can somehow support and enhance the creative process, we must then (1) specify *which* features of the state account for its claimed beneficial effects and (2) explain *how* they bring about these effects. Next, I identify two potentially advantageous features of oceanic experience – unconventional perception and positive secondary affect – and explain their benefits in terms of undifferentiated low-level vision and affective elevation/support, respectively.

Undifferentiated perception

Fusion states can involve rather peculiar ways of perceiving things. Ehrenzweig, too, was struck by this fact – so much so, in fact, that he built his theory of artistic creativity around it (Ehrenzweig, 1953, 1967).

Contemporaneous psychoanalytic studies had mostly sought to unearth the unconscious conflicts, wishes, and fantasies embedded in art. By contrast, Ehrenzweig opted to examine the structural and perceptual aspects of the unconscious mind. That is, he focused on how the mind functions *formally* in the making and experiencing of art instead of detailing the individual repressed *contents* that presumably motivated and became manifest in and through these processes.

As outlined earlier, Ehrenzweig's theory holds that the mind as structured into surface and depth levels, both of which incorporate distinct modes of attention and perception. Differentiated surface-level attention produces consciously controlled, narrowly focused, and distinctly articulated perception, whereas undifferentiated depth-level attention produces unconscious, fluid, diffuse, and holistic perception. Unconscious imagery is habitually withdrawn from conscious perception – not just because of its offensive content, but because of its undifferentiated structure. Ehrenzweig calls this mechanism "purely formal 'structural' repression" (1967, p. 32).

On these grounds, Ehrenzweig argues that authentic artistic creativity requires extensive use of depth-level perception. Why should this be so? Basically, Ehrenzweig regards painting (and art-making in general) as an open-ended process of discovery: as an uncertain and oft-surprising relationship of mutual give and take. Simply put, it is not a mechanical process that merely seeks to transfer preconceived ideas or images into the final work. That being the case, painting requires from the artist the capacity to manage a profusion of options and the ability to make decisions without exact knowledge of end results. According to Ehrenzweig, this is where the depth mind's low-level vision plays a crucial functional role. He maintains that, even though it may appear vague and chaotic from the viewpoint of surface perception, undifferentiated low-level vision is in fact a *superior perceptual tool*. First, its conjunctive and syncretistic scanning dispenses with the dominant compulsion to see things in terms of separations and opposites (such as inside versus outside, figure versus ground). This free intermixing of imagery serves to boost unconventional and non-habitual symbol formation. Second, due to its wide perceptual range, low-level vision gathers information effectively and comprehensively, which in turn enables the artist to tie disparate visual elements together in the space of the work. With the aid of undifferentiated vision, then, the artist can simultaneously perceive the relations between all parts of the painting and grasp its overall compositional structure – even while working on one specific part only (Ehrenzweig, 1967, pp. 32–46). Newton echoes Ehrenzweig's observations:

> Strange though it may seem . . . this unconscious mode of operation, devoid of the reflection and contemplation of more rational consciousness, has a far greater capacity to cope with and organise a complex scenario appearing incomprehensible to the conscious mind.
>
> (2008, p. 39)

Thus, by disrupting the fixity and rigidity of habitual surface perception, low-level vision enables the painter (1) to manage the open-endedness, complexity, and uncertainty of creative work and (2) to combine undifferentiated imagery into new and vital formations.

Ehrenzweig links undifferentiated perception directly to oceanic experience by marking out a "manic-oceanic phase" in the creative cycle (1967, p. 103). This phase is initiated by a gradual descent into depth-level perception or, as Ehrenzweig describes it, by an active and deliberate surrender to the "pull of the deep" (p. 196). As attention gradually sinks towards the depths of the mind, a near-oceanic limit approaches, and once the deepest level is reached, undifferentiated oceanic perception suffuses the surface mind. Again, in this state there is an unlimited mutual interpenetration between images and objects: opposites are undone, inner and outer worlds merge, and the restrictions of space and time are dissolved (pp. 103, 120, 192). In effect, all splitting and choice making is temporarily suspended. On a similar note, psychoanalyst David Werman states that in the oceanic state, "the artist transcends the laws of constancy and is able to discern new or latent forms in objects; he seeks out hidden qualities that are not apparent in the more accessible schemata of things" (1986, p. 136). The expected payoff is substantial: "In this 'manic' stage all accidents seem to come right; all fragmentation is resolved" (Ehrenzweig, 1967, p. 103). In short, it is in those very moments when the painter feels merged with the painting that depth-level perception operates most profitably.

It is remarkable how similar the mentioned perceptual shifts in artistic creativity are to those experienced in certain types of contemplative meditation. In several studies conducted by Deikman (1963, 1966), meditators were asked to describe their perceptual reactions to a designated object, namely, a blue vase. Although the extent of perceptual changes varied between subjects, four common reactions emerged (Deikman, 1966, p. 331). First, the meditators reported an increased vividness and richness in their perceptions of the vase. Second, the vase appeared to become animated, even seeming to move as if it had a life of its own. Third, there was a notable decrease in self–object distinction, especially in those meditators who continued longest in the experiments. One subject described it thus: "I really began to feel, you know, almost as though the blue and I were perhaps merging, or that vase and I were. . . . It was as though everything was sort of merging" (p. 331). Finally, the meditators also reported syncretistic thinking and an alteration in, and fusing of, normal perceptual modes. More recent studies on perceptual change and self-boundary dissolution in meditative/mystical experience lend credence to the basic gist of these findings (see, e.g., Andersen, Schjoedt, Nielbo, & Sørensen, 2014; Ataria, 2014; Ataria, Dor-Ziderman, & Berkovich-Ohana, 2015; Millière, Carhart-Harris, Roseman, Trautwein, & Berkovich-Ohana, 2018; Lindahl & Britton, 2019).

To borrow Deikman's terminology, both artistic and meditative perceptual shifts and the concomitant feelings of merger are attributable to *de-automatization*. This means that in both cases,

> the pragmatic systems of automatic selection are set aside or break down, in favor of alternate modes of consciousness whose stimulus processing may be less efficient from a biological point of view but whose very inefficiency may permit the experience of aspects of the real world formerly excluded or ignored.
>
> (1966, pp. 337–338)

Shifting back to Ehrenzweig's perspective, we might say that undifferentiated perception may indeed be inefficient for the pragmatic purposes of biological survival but can still work very efficiently for other purposes – especially artistic creativity.

Let us suppose that the preceding is essentially correct: that in the oceanic state the object/painting can really look different, and how it looks can aid the creative process. Even if this is the case, undifferentiated oceanic perception does not *by itself* guarantee good artistic solutions or, for that matter, any creative outcomes at all. At least two further conditions need to be met for this to happen. First, there must be fruitful interplay between depth-level and surface-level processing, and second, the subject must put this interchange to use for artistically creative purposes. With respect to the first requirement, Ehrenzweig repeatedly underlines the fact that art-making consists in *cyclic oscillation* between undifferentiated and differentiated perception. Surrendering to depth perception for creative support does not mean falling back on some kind of automatic functioning wherein conscious control and choice making are forfeited altogether. The aim is instead to achieve a flexible ego rhythm in which both modes play an important role (Ehrenzweig, 1967, pp. 95–110). Marion Milner – who worked together with Ehrenzweig to discern the psychodynamics of artistic creativity – likewise highlights the role in art-making of the mind's "porpoise-like movement": its emergence and submergence between surface and depth perception (1987, p. 242).

All in all, I find Ehrenzweig's and Milner's views on oscillation fundamentally sound. However, there is some ambiguity as to what the suggested 'porpoise-like' movement consists in. Townsend, for instance, interprets the two theorists as regarding "the artist's process as an alternation between two very different states of mind" and thus to be suggesting that, "at any one moment, the artist is *either* in one mode *or* the other" (2019, p. 54, emphasis in original). In contrast to this presumed position, Townsend argues that the artist is "*both* at one with the developing work *and* able to focus on details, although one or the other state will be to the fore at any particular moment" (p. 56, emphasis in original). To elucidate this matter, I suggest a clearer distinction between mental *states* and *modes*. A state of mind is the particular mental condition that a subject is in at a specific time. A mode, in turn, is a specific way in which something is experienced, expressed, or processed. In my understanding, Ehrenzweig suggests that surface and depth *modes* are necessarily simultaneously present in all experience, and therefore also intertwined in all mental states. It is the *extent* or *degree* to which one or the other mode is emphasized that will determine, for example, how we perceive our surroundings in any given mental state. I therefore contend that the oceanic state is a unitary state of mind in which two mental modes – 'surface' and 'depth', or, in Deikman's terms, 'action' and 'receptive' – intermix in a distinctive, characteristic way. To put this more precisely, the oceanic state is characterized by an overall accentuation or dominance of the undifferentiated depth mode. This does not mean that in oceanic experience the surface mode is, or needs to be, completely relinquished. It is only when a certain threshold of relatively stable differentiation is reached that it is no longer sensible to speak of the experiential state as 'oceanic'. From this point of view, there can be oscillation between surface and depth modes *within* the oceanic state, but only if this occurs in a way that preserves the latter mode's sufficient hold on experience. I believe that this explication not only clears Townsend's concern but is also compatible with Ehrenzweig's and Milner's views on the matter.

So, the first precondition for the artistic benefit of undifferentiated perception is that it be brought into fruitful interplay with surface-level processing. The second precondition is that this interchange be *put to use* for specifically creative purposes. This indicates that oceanic dedifferentiation and cyclic oscillation can be deliberately pursued and actively utilized to achieve different kinds of aims. There are, of course, various factors that play into whether the oceanic state is achieved and how it is exploited (if it is at all). As Deikman says of de-automatization, "the extent to which such a shift takes place is a function of the *motivation* of the individual, his particular *neurophysiological state*, and the *environmental conditions* encouraging or discouraging such a change" (1966, p. 338, my italics). To these factors we might add the *methodical practice* and *acquired skills* of the individual. Indeed, Ehrenzweig's art pedagogy rests on the very notion of learning how to avail oneself of depth perception. He discusses how surface-level perception can be willfully disrupted and suffused into depth-level processing, and also reflects on how to deal with the anxiety that this might provoke (1967, p. 212). The ultimate aim of artistic growth is a more flexible and creative ego – one that is more tolerant of uncertainty and ambiguity.

On the whole, the deliberate use of undifferentiated perception for creative purposes can be seen as separating the artist's oceanic experience from various other kinds of oceanic states. Milner expresses this idea outright:

> But it is not the oceanic feeling by itself, for that would be the mystic's state; it is rather the oceanic state in a cyclic oscillation with the activity of what Ehrenzweig calls the surface mind. . . . [A]nd the cyclic oscillation is not just passively experienced but actively used, with the *intent to make something, produce something*.
>
> (1987, p. 197, my italics)

Whether or not all states of mystical fusion are categorically lacking in creative aims may be up for debate; for artistically productive oceanic states such aims are, however, a necessity.

To sum up, undifferentiated oceanic perception can (in cyclic oscillation with surface perception) benefit artistic creativity in at least the following ways: (1) it can liberate the artist from rigid, habitual, and sterile ways of seeing things and thus enable novel and vital symbol formation; (2) it can provide an efficient and comprehensive means for gathering visual information and thus enable the artist to better grasp the overall structure of her work; and (3) in supporting the perception of several options at once, it can enable the artist to hold on to disparate visual elements and to tie them together in the pictorial space of the work. Together, these three perceptual features support the painter in managing the complexity, open-endedness, and uncertainty of much creative work.

Affective elevation and support

In addition to providing perceptual support, oceanic states can buttress the creative process affectively. To reiterate, I have discussed oceanic feelings as feelings of self-boundary dissolution and/or fusion. In addition to these primary affective features, oceanic states often involve a host of other, *secondary* affects. Ecstasy, mania, bliss, emancipation, well-being, connectedness, transcendence, tranquility, harmony, sublimity, and vitality are among the most frequently mentioned positive secondary feelings (Ehrenzweig, 1967; Storr, 1989; Fauteux, 1995; Rooney, 2007; Comte-Sponville, 2008). On the flip side, the oceanic feeling has been noted to induce negative affects ranging from fear of drowning and "losing one's hold on the solid earth" to overwhelming dread and horror of annihilation (Milner, 1957, p. 24; Harrison, 1986). Strictly speaking, these secondary affects are contingent and therefore non-essential features of the oceanic feeling. It is therefore more accurate to say that oceanic states often give rise to, or are accompanied by, such affects, and that these affects in turn contribute to the overall experience in which the oceanic feeling plays a crucial part.

The valence and intensity of the secondary affects depend on a variety of factors, including the expectations, beliefs, judgments, and overall psychological disposition of the subject; the social, cultural, and historical context in which the state emerges and unfolds; and the nature of the fused-with object. As mentioned, feelings of fusion can engender considerable anxiety. Especially in psychosis, "oceanic dedifferentiation is felt and feared as death itself" (Ehrenzweig, 1967, p. 122). According to Ehrenzweig, this is because the psychotic mind lacks the capacity to safely carry out the cycle in which elements of surface perception are dissolved, reshaped, and readmitted back into consciousness. The fragmented psychotic ego is unable to rely on oceanic depth perception to produce cohesive and meaningful symbols; all that lurks beneath its fragile surface is uncontrollable chaos or emptiness (Ehrenzweig, 1967, pp. 123–125). In contrast to this, the sufficiently strong and flexible ego can tolerate and put to good use the temporary dissolution of its surface functions. If the oceanic state occurs within these parameters, it is more likely to entail positive secondary feelings. For example, Newton recounts that he "was not in any way fearful of drowning, being overwhelmed or lost" during his oceanic state; "rather the experience was to be expected and welcomed" (2008, p. 50). To amplify this positive overtone, Newton also describes oceanic experience as a "safety net" that protects, supports, and carries forward the creative process. Falling back on this net, he continues, is accompanied by feelings of elation, ecstasy, and magical control (p. 71, pp. 84–87).

Ehrenzweig likewise highlights the positive affective profile of oceanic experience. As the term '*manic*-oceanic phase' reveals, he pays particular heed to its intensely elevated affective quality. On the one hand, Ehrenzweig considers such manic feelings as reverberations of the descent into the oceanic level of the depth mind. He writes: "Dedifferentiation suspends many kinds of boundaries and distinctions; at an extreme limit it may remove the boundaries of individual existence and so produce a mystic oceanic feeling that is distinctly manic in quality" (1967, p. 294). On the other hand, he speculates whether it is not the removal of boundaries *per se* that produces the manic feelings, but rather the rising into conscious awareness of the *products* of dedifferentiated perception (p. 295). Either way, Ehrenzweig asserts that the manic quality of oceanic dedifferentiation can serve to protect and sustain creativity. As he puts it, "a manic element belonging to deeper near-oceanic levels of dedifferentiation (where unconscious scanning is carried on) must persist to sustain the artist against the onslaught of depression at the sight of persisting surface fragmentation" (1967, p. 193). In this account, the oceanic state not only comprises a valuable mode of perception but also provides an *affective safeguard* against the perturbation and uncertainty caused by the creative process. In this way, manic fusion serves an important constructive role in artistic work.

Moreover, the elevated mood of oceanic states can enhance the artist's positive feelings about the *developing painting itself*. In the manic-oceanic state the developing work can feel exceptionally significant and vital – as an object that is worth all the hard work being put into its creation. At best, the painting can strike the artist as exceedingly spectacular – as good as perfect – which may in turn evoke in the artist feelings of grandiosity and omnipotence. This bears witness to the fact that, in the state of merger, the detached, critical, and analytical form of evaluation has been temporarily suspended. Viewed from this perspective, it is "not difficult to see how the oceanic experience can play an incisive role in creative activity, particularly where feelings of awe, vastness, solemnity, high-purpose, or intense love *pervade the artistic product*" (Werman, 1986, p. 136, my italics).

Finally, besides safeguarding creativity and boosting the apparent worth of one's work (and one's self), elevated affect can play a *guiding* role in the artistic process (see Collingwood, 1958; Anderson & Hausman, 1992; Nelson & Rawlings, 2007). Based on interviews with professional artists, Barnaby Nelson and David Rawlings found that highness of mood was experienced as not only propelling the artistic activity forward but also as directing the course of the work. It can indicate to the artist that her artwork is progressing well and in the right direction, encouraging her to continue in a manner which maintains this mood (Nelson & Rawlings, 2007, p. 232). In terms of affective scaffolding, then, the oceanic state can be said to engender and sustain a positive, elevated mood, which in turn may scaffold the creative process by signaling whether it is progressing in a satisfactory direction.

Concluding remarks

In this chapter, I have examined how painting can scaffold feelings of self-boundary dissolution and fusion with paintings-in-progress. In essence, these oceanic experiences embody the fundamental existential concern of relating subjective and objective reality and demarcating between self and not-self. Moreover, I have argued that painters may come to value oceanic states for two main reasons. First, oceanic experience foregrounds a mode of undifferentiated perception that can be used to manage the complexity of artistic creativity and to enhance novel symbol formation. Second, it typically involves positive secondary affects that can serve to protect, vitalize, and guide the creative process.

A considerable proportion of my analysis has relied on Ehrenzweig's writings on art and creativity. Certainly, his theorization provides a substantial selection of tools to anatomize the perceptual and affective features of artistic work. Even so, there are areas in his thinking that give rise to critical questions and concerns. First of all, Ehrenzweig tends to use rather high-flown language to describe oceanic experiencing. This loftiness might divert attention from its more mitigated and arguably more common instantiations in everyday artistic creativity. Second, he does not explicate in sufficient detail the ties between oceanic depth perception and actual artistic symbol formation. How, precisely, is visual material chosen and extracted from the flow of undifferentiated low-level vision to produce new imagery within the developing painting? (For a similar concern, see Wright, 1998, p. 79.) Finally, I find Ehrenzweig's proclamation that depth perception is a necessary precondition of "authentic" artistic creativity to be problematically normative (1967, pp. 228–229). Does all vital and significant art really need to rely on oceanic low-level vision in the proposed sense? Taking this position would effectively exclude from 'authentic' art a considerable amount of products, the making of which cannot plausibly be said to have incorporated depth-level perception but which nonetheless could be considered highly creative and aesthetically valuable objects. In short, I do not find it plausible to posit the employment of oceanic perception as a universal criterion for the 'authenticity' of artistic creativity, nor for the value of the works produced therein. In order to distance myself from this normative stance, I simply maintain that recourse to an oceanic phase or state in creativity is but *one possible* element of artistic creativity.

All of this is not to negate the existence or potential significance of oceanic perception and feeling in artistic creativity, but rather to present a more tempered approach to it. Seeing as painters paint for different reasons and in different ways, I do not wish to give the impression that all painting necessarily involves, or indeed needs to involve, oceanic experience in the specified perceptual-affective sense. As stated previously, I do not wish to make any universal or normative claims about the essence of artistic creativity. That being said, I do believe that many painters experience feelings of the oceanic kind in relation to their paintings. Thus, my more moderate view is that under certain conditions painting can scaffold oceanic experience, and that this experience can in turn affect painting in various beneficent ways. There is something rather appealing about the possibility of honing one's perceptual skills to see things more vividly and deeply than habit allows. Simply put, the prospect of broadening one's perceptual and aesthetic sensibilities to include oceanic low-level scanning is a truly alluring option. In this view, painters can explore and learn to use oceanic depth-level perception to advance their artistic work. For some, it might turn out to be a crucially valuable find.

Chapter 6

Getting it right

Of all the feelings scaffolded by painting, one in particular seems to stand out for artists. In the words of painter Luc Tuymans, "the most important thing in painting is when it works out. When you're doing it you can *feel the moment when something is correct*. There's also a particular joy of doing it; it's very physical, and it's fairly conscious" (Tuymans, 2005, my italics). Agnes Martin, in turn, tells of the often-difficult process of finding out what works in painting:

> Something tells you that you *haven't* yet painted what you must paint. Then, when you finally paint what you're supposed to paint, then something tells you "OK, this is *it*!". If you accept a painting with good points, but isn't really *it*, then you're not on the track. You're permanently derailed. It's through discipline and tremendous disappointment and failure that you arrive at what it is you must paint.
>
> (Gruen, 1991, pp. 83–84, emphasis in original)

Finally, on much the same note, Richard Diebenkorn reflects:

> Now the idea is to get everything right – it's not just color or form or line – it's everything all at once. Of course, that doesn't work either, so it's a continuous struggle. Sometimes you sail along. When I'm halfway there with a painting, it can occasionally be thrilling, and I can stop and say, "Gee, how lucky I am to be doing this activity that I like to do!" But it happens very rarely, usually it's agony.
>
> (Gruen, 1991, p. 63)

When achieved, the sense of correctness is often accompanied by various other pleasurable feelings, such as vitalization, self-cohesion, and perfection. All of this suggests that the rightness of one's paintings is not just a matter of dispassionate perception or judgment but, in a pivotal way, something that is *felt*.

In this chapter, I delve deeper into the feeling of getting a painting to work. I maintain that this feeling cannot be understood in isolation from the underlying dynamics and aims of painting or from the overall creative cycle in which it occurs. For the most part, I develop my view in dialogue with two recent psychoanalytical accounts of artistic creativity, namely, those of Patricia Townsend (2019) and George Hagman (2005, 2010). Both authors draw from a relational approach to creativity and, in keeping with this, emphasize the developmentally and dyadically structured underpinnings of painting. Building on their ideas, I submit that painting constitutes a special relationship in which the painter seeks to address and give form to elements of her personal experience. From this perspective, the feeling of getting it right signals that one's experience has been satisfactorily dealt with in and through the painting. The rest of this chapter will expand on this basic claim.

The 'it' in getting it right

When we think of the feeling of getting it right, two critical questions soon emerge: (1) Under what *conditions* does a painting typically feel right? And (2) Is there something that the painting feels right *in relation* to, and in relation to which its rightness becomes *intelligible*? As I have previously underlined, painters paint in different cultural-historical contexts and with widely varying methods, styles, and aims. This makes it futile to try to identify any essential form or content that all painters seek to get right in their creative work. That crucial 'something' in relation to which a painting either achieves or fails to achieve its rightness may be the characteristic feel of a portrait sitter, an elaborate metaphysical idea, an illusory visual effect, a religious narrative, a stylistic convention, and so on and so forth. From a psychodynamic standpoint, it is apparent that there will typically be numerous factors – some more conscious than others – that determine the rightness of any given work. In this sense, feelings of rightness can be said to be *overdetermined*. Moreover, the grounds for rightness often change and develop as the creative work progresses, and may become established only after lengthy periods of trial and error.

The variable contextual determination of correctness is aptly illustrated by painter Frank Stella's response to the Abstract Expressionist art of the 1940s and 1950s. Although the artists classified under this label formed a notably heterogeneous group, many were committed to an *instinctive* and *self-expressive* style of painting. In this kind of artistic work, the feeling of rightness depends on how successfully the task of spontaneous expression is resolved during the unfolding painterly activity. That is to say, the feeling arises through responsive engagement with the painting and links back directly to the painter's experience of what is going on in the work. In contrast to this, Stella deliberately eschewed the role of immediate feeling and instinct in painting. The execution of his Minimalist *Black Paintings* (1958–1960) was instead preceded by meticulous planning. The actual activity of painting began only after he had established a clear motif and an emotionally detached mechanical method for its implementation. In this predetermined manner, Stella sought to erase all traces of individual subjectivity and human touch from the paintings and, more generally, to question the nature of painting as immediate creative expression. If Stella indeed felt his work to 'click' at any point, it was not through an interactive process of exploration and discovery played out on the canvas surface, nor did it depend primarily on what he felt while applying the paint. Compared to the Abstract Expressionists, then, his feelings of correctness were arguably of a very different kind. This goes to show that the feeling – its experiential character, its role in the creative process, and its personal significance – is fundamentally conditioned by the specific aims, methods, and artistic self-conceptions of the painter and by the overall setting in which the painting occurs.

Yet, even as we acknowledge the vast diversity of painting praxes, we might wonder whether there might still be a basic point of reference for most if not all painters' feelings of rightness. I believe that there is indeed such a basis: the artist's *own experience*. Simply put, whatever contents and forms any given painting process deals with, these are always rooted in the painter's personal perspective on the world. Revealingly, when painter David Hockney was asked about the generally *autobiographical nature* of his work, he replied:

> Yes, but all artists must deal with that, in a way. They deal with their own experience. How can you deal with something else? I mean, even if you are dealing with something else, it has to be filtered

> through your own experience and feelings. In that sense, it's always autobiographical.
>
> (Cork, 2015, p. 94)

Painter and conceptual artist Michael Craig-Martin encapsulates the same view nicely: "Works of art are the products of our attempts to give expressive form to our personal experience of the world in order to make it available to others" (2015, p. 179). Stella's *Black Paintings*, too, were 'autobiographical' in this fundamental sense. Creating the series gave form to his intellectually fleshed-out observations, deliberations, and judgments – that is, to his lived experience – of a contemporary artistic trend, Abstract Expressionism. In sum, regardless of what painting deals with, it does so in relation to the artist's experiential world.

On these grounds, I maintain that a painting feels right to its maker when *it succeeds in addressing and giving satisfactory form to some important element (or elements) of her personal experience*. By 'personal experience' I mean the variable appearance of things to an individual conscious subject. More specifically, things can be said to appear to a subject under various experiential modes or types – for example, through memory, perception, ideation, contemplation, embodied action, feeling, desire, intuition, wish, fantasy, and so on. Furthermore, as both psychoanalysis and phenomenological philosophy have underlined, experience has a cumulative and sedimented structure (see Chapter 4). It is out of this vast and layered pool of past and present experience that all manner of 'elements' – ideas, intuitions, percepts, images, problems, impulses, motifs – will emerge, some of which will strike the painter as worthy of further artistic exploration. The feeling of getting it right will then hinge on the successful handling of these experiential elements in painterly form.

As it stands, this might seem like a fairly trivial and vague claim to make – a truism that does not yet tell us precisely *how* or *why* feelings of rightness occur in painting. Thus, to add more cogency to my argument, I elaborate it vis-à-vis the psychoanalytical writings of Patricia Townsend and George Hagman. Both authors argue that, in essence, painting aims to articulate the artist's inchoate inner experience. Moreover, they submit that the work of art not only mirrors subjective experience but also offers a new perspective on the external world, and can only be created through a process in which both of these aspects of reality flow into and inform one another. In line with this approach, Hagman and Townsend highlight the *special relationship* between the artist's subjective experience and the painting-in-progress. Their shared premise is that, as the painting is gradually imbued with subjective psychic material, it becomes, in Winnicottian parlance, a *subjective object* or, in the self-psychological term Hagman prefers, a *selfobject* (see Kohut, 2011). In short, the painter comes to interact with an object that contains, reorganizes, and reflects back externalized elements of her own experience. It is in this light, I argue, that the feeling of getting it right can be better understood.

However, a final qualifying note is in order before I move on to discuss the feeling of correctness with regard to Townsend's and Hagman's thinking. To keep things manageable, I again limit my examination to painting praxes that rely on synchronous and causally bidirectional interaction between the painter and the developing work. As outlined in Chapter 2, in this kind of process the artist manipulates the painting in ways that cause her to readjust her prior intentions towards that painting, which in turn prompts her to carry out further modifying actions, and so on cyclically until the work is considered complete. The following quotes from three different painters testify to the kind of painting that I have in mind. The first is from Rita Ackermann:

> I heard an artist say, "When I'm painting, I know what I am doing, but I don't know what I am making." It makes sense, right? There is some logic there if you want to listen to what the painting has to say in the process of making. It's like trying to fix a problem or tame a wild horse: you don't know where it is going to take you or how long it will take to finish.
>
> (BOMB Magazine, 139, 2017)

Francis Bacon, too, was open to chance discovery:

> You see, when I start painting, I have an idea of what I'd like to do, but generally the accidents in the paint suggest the possibilities of developing the image in a way which seems to be very much better than anything I had thought of.
>
> (Cork, 2015, p. 33)

And Frank Auerbach sums it all up:

> I mean, to do something predicted doesn't seem worth doing at all. To actually stand in front of one's canvas and render something that has

> been thought out – I don't know whether anybody does it, but it seems to me to take all the fun out of doing it.
>
> (Cork, 2015, p. 73)

This qualification excludes from my consideration all painting practices that seek to implement predetermined plans as precisely and rigidly as possible and, as such, leave little room for exploration, chance, and discovery during the act of painting. With these parameters in place, I now turn to examine how the feeling of getting it right depends on the formalization of personal experience through responsive painting. I do so first in light of Townsend's idea of a creative *pre-sense*, and then with respect to Hagman's conception of *aesthetic resonance*.

Pre-sense, ideation, and the struggle to get it right

Townsend's approach to artistic creativity is deeply rooted in both theory and practice, and as such is particularly instructive. In her book *Creative States of Mind* (2019), she draws from her own artistic expertise and from interviews with 33 other professional artists to highlight various experiential aspects of the creative process. At the same time, she uses psychoanalytical theorization – with Winnicott at the forefront – to investigate the psychodynamic mechanisms and developmental processes that underlie the discussed experiential states. In short, Townsend brings psychoanalytical theory, her own experience, and the interviews into a mutual conversation that applies and refines the distinctive contributions of each source to the understanding of art-making.

According to Townsend, the creative process begins with the emergence of a *pre-sense*: a pressing feeling that a new work of art could be, or indeed *must* be, created (2019, pp. 6–16). In her view, this pre-sense arises when an element of the outside world stirs something in the artist's inner experience, which in turn calls for its further exploration and subsequent formalization in artwork. In short, a pre-sense is a vague and stimulating hunch rather than a clear idea for a work of art. In this indefiniteness, Townsend argues, pre-sensing is similar to the primary creativity of the infant (p. 10). To reiterate, in primary creativity the infant searches for something to meet his needs (without knowing what this could be) and illusorily creates this 'something' just as the caregiver turns up to satisfy him (see Chapter 3). Townsend traces a "direct line" from this early experience to the use of a transitional object, to older children's play, and finally, to artistic creativity: "The artist too has an intimation (a pre-sense) that there is something to be found or, rather, created that will correspond with an inner experience (whether or not she eventually succeeds in creating such a form)" (p. 10). To be clear, Townsend does not *equate* mature artistic practice with infantile creativity or children's play. She duly points out that art is made "within a cultural context, drawing on a cultural heritage and usually with the intention of presenting the finished work to an audience" (p. 10). Moreover, in art-making, a new object is *actually* created – not just imagined or played with.

I find the concept of 'pre-sense' useful as it is. That said, I want to clarify a couple of things before discussing it with respect to the feeling of getting it right. As mentioned, Townsend singles out *perceptions of the outside world* as the main triggers for a pre-sense (2019, pp. 6–16). Moreover, when she suggests that "something 'out there' . . . *resonates* with something inner", she appears to identify a rudimentary sense of rightness at this early stage of the creative process (p. 12, my italics). Overall, this implies two things: first, that artistic creativity is mainly, if not exclusively, inspired by something that is discovered in one's external surroundings, and second, that whatever is thus discovered instigates further artistic exploration because it is felt to match with some important element(s) of one's inarticulate inner experience. While the first claim may often hold true, I find it tends to diminish the significance of the artist's *inner world* in instigating a pre-sense. To give just one counterexample, fantasies and reveries often give rise to a pressing need to create art. Although the contents of such imaginings may be connected to the outside world, it would be counterintuitive to maintain that, in this case, the pre-sense originates from a current or recent perception of the external world. As regards the second claim, I certainly agree that a rudimentary sense of inner-outer resonance can inspire artistic work. But I also wonder whether this kind of resonance is absolutely necessary, considering that an artistic pre-sense can quite demonstrably derive from an elemental sense of *dissonance*, as well – for example, from a conflict between one's desires and morals or a tension between what one sees and what one wishes to see.

Thus, to balance out the picture, I submit that a creative pre-sense usually emerges from elements of both inner and outer reality *together*, with one or the other possibly being emphasized in any given case. I also suggest that a pre-sense can be established by discord rather than inner-outer resonance. Frank Auerbach's reflections on his artistic motives aptly demonstrate the complexity of this matter. He observes: "One has a life, and the people one is involved with seem to me tremendously worth recording. There are these people whom one pays attention to, who will never occur again" (Cork, 2015, p. 68). Based solely on this, we might assume that Auerbach's creative pre-sensing depends predominantly on the perception of the external world – specifically, of other people. But he goes on to add:

> I think people do start painting because a sort of *anxiety about time*. One knows that the experience is going to go, one knows the people are going to disappear, so one tries to pin them down. . . . There has to be a sort of *conflict* between what one wants and what actually exists.
> (p. 68, my italics)

This indicates that the pre-sensing crucial to his work is equally generated by significant internal pressures and concerns.

Regardless of how a particular pre-sense takes hold, it needs to be developed into a more specific, workable idea (Townsend, 2019, pp. 17–26). Different artists apply different methods to make this happen. Townsend notes that, in general, there are two possible approaches available. While some artists prefer to engage with their chosen medium immediately, others make various preparations – for example, by researching their subject matter or by producing preliminary sketches and studies (p. 16). Once the idea becomes clearer, the artist typically feels elated and energized. Often, the illumined idea is held in idealized regard: it feels like a perfect fit with the pre-sense that prompted the creative exploration (pp. 27–36). Here we can definitely discern an incipient feeling of getting the work right or, at least, of getting it on the *right track*. However, as Townsend points out, the impression of an ideal fit between one's pre-sense, the idea, and the embryonic artwork tends to be short-lived. When the actual hands-on manipulation of the medium progresses, the artist will inevitably encounter frustrating challenges and disappointing limitations. The sense of perfection will then give way to a more realistic appraisal of the idea's possible realization (pp. 37–39).

In her study, Townsend details the various ways in which artists engage with their media to bring their ideas to final fruition. Like many other relationally oriented writers, she characterizes the creative process as a dialogue in which the work responds to the gestures of the artist and leads the interaction into new and unexpected territory. And, in line with Winnicottian thinking, she considers this artistic exchange to parallel early infant–caregiver engagements. Put broadly, both are dyadic relationships wherein the subject seeks cohesive form for inner experience through a responsive, malleable, and mirroring external medium (Townsend, 2019, pp. 41–45). While these ideas are compelling and important, there is no need to review them any further here (see Chapter 3 for an in-depth discussion). Instead, I want to pick out for closer inspection Townsend's *own* struggle to get an obstinate work to feel right.

To start off this personal account, Townsend tells us of her fascination with a bay landscape that she witnessed undergoing rapid tidal changes (2019, pp. 61–64). In order to formalize this experience artistically, she first set out to create a two-dimensional, blue-and-ochre text-based print. However, after a "long and frustrating" process of experimenting with different texts, colors, and fonts, she thought it better to rework the piece completely as an animation instead (p. 62). But, equipped with this new medium, Townsend still failed to achieve the desired effect of a shifting tide. Following another "tortuous process" of trial and error, she finally discovered the right arrangement for her work: a three-dimensional "mountain range" of sand on which to project the animation (p. 63). This, she reflects, created a close-enough match between her inner experience – that is, her impression of the landscape – and the external work.

On the whole, then, Townsend portrays her creative process as a series of experimentations that either brought her closer to or distanced her from the specific experience she wanted to embody in the work. She recollects,

> If something did not "feel right", I was disappointed and frustrated, and I had to tolerate these feelings too, not knowing whether or not another way forward would emerge. . . . I played with different forms, transferring my experience from one to the next until I was satisfied that I had found the closest possible "fit".
>
> (2019, pp. 63–64)

Townsend relates how she assessed the changing work's fittingness on different levels of consciousness simultaneously. As she puts it, "[i]n trying out different configurations, I was assessing each variation not only in terms of whether or not it satisfied criteria of which I was aware but also whether it 'felt right' at a less conscious level" (p. 61). This indicates that feelings of rightness are, as mentioned, overdetermined: their emergence and intelligibility is accounted for by multiple factors, some of which are more conscious than others. Townsend suggests that these factors may even include residual infantile affects that are never fully accessible to conscious awareness (p. 120) – a state of affairs that testifies to the vastness and depth of our sedimented experience.

Most painters are more than familiar with these types of struggles and, like Townsend, have attested to the necessity of painstaking experimentation in finding out what feels right. Consider, for instance, David Lynch's musings on ideation and discovery:

> The idea just needs to be enough to get you started, because, for me, whatever follows is a process of action and reaction. It's always a process of building and then destroying. And then, out of this destruction, discovering a thing and building on it.
>
> (2006, p. 12)

Similarly, painter Tarja Pitkänen-Walter asserts that the most important and energizing moment in artistic work is when the painting presents its maker with something unexpected. This 'unknown' must then be followed and cultivated with the appropriate painterly gestures. However, this by itself is not enough: the unpredictable must 'grow alongside' something that has already been planned and feels familiar to the artist. In short, the painter must willingly make space for a dialogue between the unexpected and the preconceived, without allowing one to overpower the other (Saarinen, 2012b, pp. 272–276). Thus, like Lynch and Townsend, Pitkänen-Walter indicates that her artistic work incorporates a prior process of pre-sensing and ideation in relation to which something surprising may emerge and develop.

Leon Kossoff and Frank Auerbach have also talked about the challenges of getting a painting to work (see Gayford, 2018, pp. 136, 266). They both believe that, if painting is to succeed, the artist must "go beyond the familiar, beyond what is already known, into a place where he does not know what he is doing" (p. 136). In Kossoff's words, "[n]othing really begins to happen in a painting until you reach the point where conscious intention breaks up and ceases to be the thing that's driving you" (p. 266). In his experience, this turning point can be reached only via repeated error and experimentation. Auerbach also values the unpredictability that is characteristic of painting. But he makes it clear that unexpectedness does not automatically lead to success: "To have done something that one hadn't foreseen – by itself – would simply seem to be a gesture" (Cork, 2015, p. 73).

For a proper sense of rightness to emerge, at least two more conditions need to be met. First, the work must feel *true*. As Auerbach observes, "to have done something that one hadn't foreseen, but at the same time actually seems true to a specific fact, seems to me to be very exciting" (Cork, 2015, p. 73). Kossoff, too, remarks that he must continuously destroy "images that lie" (Gayford, 2018, p. 136). In line with my earlier discussion, I submit that the work feels right when it is true to certain facts about *one's own experience*. Second, in addition to being truthful, a good painting must feel *vital*. Auerbach confirms that there are "certain [truthful] configurations on canvas that feel organic and alive and quivering, and others that seem inert" (p. 136). Hence, for him, "a good painting is always a bit of a miracle" (p. 136). Taken together, these artists' reflections indicate that, in painting, feelings of correctness typically arise from absorbing yet arduous processes of open-ended exploration, and cannot be summoned up in fully preconceived and exclusively conscious fashion.

Let us pause here to recap the key points of the present discussion. Basically, Townsend argues that artistic creativity externalizes and reorganizes elements of the artist's inchoate experience through a progressive cycle of pre-sense, ideation, responsive experimentation, readjustment, and gradual completion of the work. Feelings of rightness can accordingly be seen to occur at various different stages of this process: first, when the crucial pre-sense is induced by a rudimentary sense of (inner-outer) resonance; second, when there is a fit between the pre-sense and the more specific idea for a work; third, when the pre-sense–idea compound becomes more and more truthfully articulated in the developing work; and finally, when the cycle from pre-sense to satisfactory formalization is complete and the work is considered to be finished. Ideally, when the artwork is complete, it will not only embody the artist's inner experience but also be accessible to others. It may then be 'sent out into the world' to achieve wider relevance and appeal (Townsend, 2019, pp. 99–111). Painter Howard Hodgkin captures the essence of this final stage succinctly:

> To me, a picture is really finished when, in theory at least, it's as far away from me as it would be from anyone else. So that the emotion – which is often extremely intense, the subject of the situation, the situation – becomes so *completely turned into an object*, a thing, in other words a painting, that I look at it as a painting that is being transformed. And I should be able to look at it with the same surprise and interest as anyone else.
>
> (Cork, 2015, p. 85, my italics)

In sum, as the work detaches from the artist's experience and gains independence, it can begin its second life as a publicly shared object.

Of course, painting does not need to follow a neat path from pre-sense and ideation to experimentation, readjustment, and finalization. In some cases there seems to be no real difference between pre-sense, ideation, and experimentation. Consider, for example, Gillian Ayres's style of painting. In short, her method was highly improvisatory. As Gayford describes it: "There was no blueprint, no preliminary ideas worked out in advance. . . . In the event she took, as [Jackson] Pollock did, an initial leap and then started from the way – partly chance – the pigment had fallen" (Gayford, 2018, pp. 172–173). After throwing the paints and turpentines all over the surface, "there came contemplation, adjustment, additions and subtractions" (p. 172). In this case, there is arguably no *prior* experiential pre-sense based on which the work is developed and in relation to which it can achieve its correctness. Rather, the primary conditions for rightness arise in and through the very act of painting itself. This way of painting, Ayres has revealed, is a process of "evolving something, rather in the way perhaps that a bar of music or a line of poetry follows from the last, developing and changing" (p. 173). In essence, it relies on both chance and intuitive action. To emphasize the role of the latter, Ayres refers to tennis: "You can suddenly sense that you are going to make a shot better than you usually do, and then you can't do it again" (p. 173). The point of this example is to re-emphasize that I am not seeking any blanket descriptions of creativity that are applicable across all times and cases. That said, I believe Ayres's case supports the view that feelings of rightness are necessarily tied to how personal experience is dealt with in painting – it only diminishes the significance of *prior* pre-sensing and planning and emphasizes the here and now. I will now turn to Hagman's account of painterly creativity to analyze several further important dimensions of feelings of correctness.

Selfobject experience and aesthetic resonance

Hagman shares with Townsend the fundamental view that painting seeks to give form to inchoate personal experience. However, he applies somewhat different terminology and stresses different things in analyzing the dynamic underpinnings, characteristic phases, and ulterior aims of painting. Basically, when the painter paints, she participates in a dialogue with her own subjectivity as it is being objectified in the work of art. In Hagman's terms, the artist engages with a *selfobject* of her own creation (2005, p. 79). From this perspective, painting aims at a special type of experience, namely, a *selfobject experience* in which the painting mirrors elements of one's subjectivity as satisfyingly as possible (Hagman, 2005, pp. 5–6; see also Kohut, 2011; Rotenberg, 1988). However, Hagman is quick to point out that mere self-expression does not suffice in bringing about optimal experiential outcomes. Instead, when subjectivity is expressed in painting, it needs to be expressed in *ideal form* – that is, in a way that mirrors experience as *truthfully* and *perfectly* as possible (2005, pp. 71–72). As Hagman puts it:

> We feel excited by the appearance of this ideal form. We are entranced, in awe, fascinated by its perfection, its balance, its rhythm, its color, shape, and texture. Its meanings are exquisite, complex, and resonant with our most unconscious knowledge. We are eager to engage it, to get close; we have an urge to make it part of us.
>
> (p. 60)

Hagman considers this selfobject dynamic to be rooted in early ontogenesis and argues that the "need to idealize" is a key driving force behind our (primary) attachments to other people (2005, p. 47). To be more specific, infant–caregiver interactions involve a kind of "shared idealization" in which there is "mutual pleasure, excitement, and joy at the sight of each other, the thrill of touching and vocalizing", and so on (p. 47). Importantly, in these positively attuned interchanges, both interactants value each other and thus *feel themselves to be valued* (p. 49). In this way, idealization is layered into our experiencing from early on, which in turn has us desiring the proximity of idealized objects all through life. As Hagman puts it,

> as the tendency to idealize is extended beyond the early relational context, it becomes a source of motivation to seek out, create, and engage with objects and experiences that are highly valued and gratifying, such as in the production and/or enjoyment of art.
>
> (p. 48)

This means that we continuously seek objects that mirror our subjectivity in ideal form, and by making art we attempt to create such objects for ourselves. In this way, painting can scaffold selfobject experiences that the artist may have previously been deprived of and is currently unable to attain through any other means. Indeed, for some individuals, artistic creativity may become the primary or only way to achieve these self-enhancing states.

Creating idealized selfobjects through art tends to be a demanding and uncertain affair. In Hagman's account, there are several nonlinear and frequently overlapping phases in this process (2005, pp. 73–79). In relevant respects, his portrayal of the opening stages of creativity parallels that of Townsend's account. To put it briefly, starting a painting can feel like an opportunity and a risk – both inspiring and unsettling at the same time. For the artist, each painting is initially a 'stranger' that she must gradually become acquainted with. As the work begins to feel like a partner-in-dialogue, it opens up certain opportunities and directions while closing down others. At the same time, it may feel resistant to the artist's conscious intentions and may respond to her painterly gestures in various unexpected ways – not even experienced painters are capable of fully anticipating the outcomes of this precarious interaction. However, unpredictability is generally considered to be advantageous, as it opens up space for new and surprising elements to emerge. The painter must then bring together the planned and the unpredictable to work towards a painting that reflects her experience as truthfully as possible.

The next phase of the creative process is marked by an increased sense of compatibility between the artist's subjectivity and the developing painting. Hagman describes this situation as follows:

> Here the feeling that the artwork is beginning to take form excites the artist. There is an increased experience of self-cohesion, effectiveness,

> and vitality. The artist feels in tune with the artwork, and there is a sense of resonance in which the piece seems to become a perfect reflection of the artist's inner fantasy life.
>
> (2005, p. 74)

This phase culminates in *aesthetic resonance*: an intensely pleasurable selfobject experience wherein the painting reflects its maker's subjectivity in both ideal and sufficiently truthful form (pp. 5, 74–79; Hagman, 2010, pp. 28–31). It is, as Hagman describes it, "the most affectively charged moment of the creative experience" (2005, p. 75). From a relational-developmental perspective, aesthetic resonance can be seen to derive from primary infant–caregiver attunements. Indeed, Hagman asserts that ideal form evokes the "earliest, most archaic qualities of enthrallment with the essential other", which, he concludes, "is a feeling of relatedness without comparison" (p. 60).

Frank Auerbach seems to be touching on this type of experience when he says that "there is a sort of intimacy, excitement and confidence that comes from inhabiting the painting, and knowing exactly where everything is". There is, he continues, a "sort of magic in conjuring up a real place, a record of it that is somewhere between one's feeling about the fact and the appearance. Well, more than appearance – substance" (Cork, 2015, p. 68). As I see it, this quote captures two important features of aesthetic resonance. First, it evinces an intensely absorbing and exciting bond between the painter and the painting. Moreover, it alludes to a sense of confidence about the painting – of knowing precisely how it 'works'. Second, when Auerbach describes how the painting performs its magic *somewhere between* his own feeling about an actual place and the appearance of that place in the substance of the painting, he is, to my mind, describing a selfobject (or subjective object) that is being played with and created in the potential space.

On the whole, I think 'resonance' is a viable term in this connection because it has a suitable double meaning. In a strictly physical sense, it refers to the reinforcement or prolongation of sound by reflection from a surface or by the synchronous vibration of a neighboring object (Oxford English Dictionary). If we take the liberty of shifting from physics to psychology and substitute 'sound' with feeling, imagination, thought, and so on, resonance can be said to occur when the painting (surface) synchronously reinforces and reflects elements of the artist's personal experience. But this is not all there is to resonance: it also signifies the power to *evoke* images, memories, emotions, and the like (Oxford English Dictionary). Viewed in this light, the state of aesthetic resonance not only reflects and strengthens elements of externalized experience but also elicits experience that goes *over and beyond* that which has been projected. In short, it opens up space for new experiential possibilities. I think Hagman alludes to this aspect of resonance when he says that "art is not simply a mirror, a representation of ourselves; it is a new creation that evokes self-experience and embodies the self-in-relation through aesthetic perfection" (2005, p. 5).

For all the effort put into achieving aesthetic resonance, it will unavoidably waver during the creative process (Hagman, 2005, pp. 76–77). In such moments, the externalized elements of the artist's subjectivity will feel dissonant and incompatible with her inner experience, and the work itself may appear detached, strange, and even repelling. According to Hagman, this disjunction can be "due to the effect of the object on the form of self-expression or to the rapid unfolding of the artist's self-experience" (p. 5). It is also affected by the refractory material qualities of the artistic medium itself; it is nigh-on impossible to completely control the behavior of paint on canvas. Crucially, how the artist responds to such breaks in resonance will decide the overall fate of the creative effort (p. 76). If fear of failure grows overly intense, the artist will be tempted to abandon the painting. For this reason, the final phase of creativity – namely, the completion of the work – requires considerable toleration of uncertainty and frustration. If all goes well, the artist will trust her own skills and competency and will continue to explore the work's possibilities with an open mind. By gradually refining the painting, the lost selfobject tie can be restored and the work "moved closer to a formal ideal" (p. 79). In this respect, Hagman's depiction calls to mind Townsend's persistent efforts to capture her experience more and more accurately and truthfully in her work.

Once a work is finished and let go, its self-enhancing effects will inevitably fade. For this reason, art-making can become highly addictive. Hagman states this outright:

> For the artist, it is never enough to sit and enjoy the fruit of his or her labor; the artist is compelled again and again to re-create a process of selfexperiencing in which he or she seeks an elusive yet powerful

> affective event. Once the object is finished, possessing a fully separate life, the artist must return to the process, the continuing search.
>
> (2005, p. 72)

Hagman specifies that the addictiveness of artistic creativity is not due to aesthetic resonance alone. Rather, the painter is drawn in and captivated by the *entire creative cycle* of ideation, exploration, resonance, uncertainty, and the final, ideal formalization of experience (p. 78). In short, "[t]he artist is driven to seek out again and again the experience of heightened, lost, and regained self-experience" (p. 77). Townsend, too, points out that artists are typically compelled to make new works of art. She maintains that, on the one hand, this owes to artists' need to participate in the vitalizing interaction afforded by painting. On the other, it is due to the perpetual desire of discovering oneself in and through one's own artwork (Townsend, 2019, pp. 108–109). However, the creative search can never be brought to a definitive close because no (amount of) artwork can ever fully capture the vast and formless inner experience underlying all creative pre-sense and ideation (pp. 120–121). Viewed in this light, painting is not something that the painter merely does: it is an overall way of being and a deep-rooted existential commitment.

Indeed, as I see it, Hagman places special emphasis on the *existential import* of ideal artistic form. Case in point, he argues that painting not only gives form to all manner of feelings, impressions, and perceptions but also externalizes the painter's subjectivity in a more comprehensive and profound way (Hagman, 2005, p. 5). In his words,

> [the] form of self-expression contained in artistic creation is best captured in the idea of *being*, of conveying in the work aspects of how it feels to be the living person whom one is. It means that the painter attempts to express in symbolic aesthetic form her *whole lived life* and *feeling of being*.
>
> (p. 5, my italics)

Successfully formalizing one's experiential life will in turn engender intense feelings of self-continuity, cohesion, and vitalization (pp. 68–79). Hagman suggests that 'self-continuity' extends beyond the sense of a stable existence to include the feeling that one's life forms a meaningful and coherent whole. Likewise, 'vitalization' surpasses mere bodily upheaval to encompass the feeling of being fully alive and open to oneself, others, and the world (pp. 74–79). In this respect, his view ties in directly with Winnicott's conception of creativity as a form of self-discovery; of achieving a unitary sense of "I AM, I am alive, I am myself" (Winnicott, 1971, pp. 53–64; see Chapter 3). It also corresponds with my view of painting as a special means to address the core concerns of personal existence.

In sum, aesthetic resonance results from the harmonious conjunction between the painter's subjective experience and its formalization in painting. In this broad sense, it is analogous to the feelings of getting it right discussed vis-à-vis Townsend's account of creativity – albeit with a specific emphasis on idealization. Moreover, if we consider paintings to embody the artist's "deepest experience of being in the world", as Hagman suggests (2005, p. 72), aesthetic resonance can be characterized as an existentially grounded feeling of getting it right. Viewed as such, it not only signals an ideal fit between the work and various elements of the artist's experience but also constitutes a more profound sense of one's overall worth – amounting, at best, to feelings of perfection and grandiosity. Perhaps such feelings are less frequent than 'regular' feelings of getting a work to click, but they are all the more powerful and desirable.

Concluding remarks

I have suggested that feelings of 'getting it right' may well be the most valued and sought-after affects scaffolded by painting. My principal premise has been that these feelings are properly intelligible only in relation to the underlying *aims* and *dynamics* of painting and to the overall *creative cycle* in which they occur. To elaborate on the first part of this proposition, I have argued that, via painting, painters essentially aim to address and give form to element(s) of their personal experience. This means that the ideas, images, problems, conflicts, etc. that both motivate painting and are worked out *in* painting arise from, and are necessarily embedded in, the artist's past and present experience. Viewed in this light, painting can indeed be said to *target* the artist's personal experiential world – regardless of its overt form and content. In making this claim, I have emphasized that 'experience' needs to be understood broadly as consisting of memory, perception, ideation, thought, embodied action, feeling, desire, intuition, fantasy, and so on. In this approach, it is not viable to single out *affect* as that which is exclusively or even primarily addressed in painting (see Chapter 3). Rather, as I have repeatedly underlined, painting is equally devoted to the articulation of highly sophisticated cognitions, acute perceptions, deeply held beliefs about what is good/virtuous/important, and so on and so forth. From this point of view, feelings of getting it right are necessarily overdetermined: their emergence and intelligibility depend on numerous conscious and unconscious elements that vary from artist to artist and from genre to genre. Even so, the sense of correctness is always grounded in and reflects the artist's own experience of the world. In sum, then, I have claimed that feelings of getting it right depend on how successfully key elements of personal experience are dealt with and formalized in the developing painting.

As regards the overall creative cycle in which feelings of rightness occur, I have restricted my examination to the kind of painting that is based on synchronous and causally bidirectional interaction between the painter and the developing work. As I have shown, this type of praxis relies heavily on exploration, experimentation, unpredictability, discovery, and readjustment. It is through an open-ended dialogical process of give and take (and trial and error) that certain experiential elements become increasingly refined and articulated in external painterly form. Feelings of rightness can accordingly be seen to occur at various stages of this cycle. Based on Townsend's account, I have suggested that they may arise, first, when a given pre-sense is induced by an elementary and exciting sense of resonance; second, when a good fit is found between the pre-sense and a more developed idea for a work; third, when the pre-sense–idea amalgam becomes more and more accurately articulated in and through the chosen medium; and finally, when the process from pre-sense to satisfactory formalization is considered to be complete. To add to this, I have drawn from Hagman's account to argue that feelings of rightness can also be understood in terms of the achievement (and wavering) of aesthetic resonance. In this view, the feeling of getting it right is a gratifying selfobject experience in which the artist feels the painting to embody her subjectivity in both ideal and truthful form. Crucially, this does not only involve the successful formalization of particular experiential elements but, in its most intense and pleasurable form, also vitalizes and enriches the artist's overall sense of being. In such cases, feelings of correctness hold considerable existential import.

Based on this, I propose that feelings of getting it right have a *dual structure*. On the one hand, they depend on and become intelligible in relation to the *specific* experiential elements that are being worked on in the painting. This aspect of correctness hinges on how well the underlying aim of addressing and formalizing certain elements of one's experiential world is fulfilled by the created work – as witnessed by Townsend's personal struggle in getting her work to click. On the other hand, feelings of rightness relate to one's subjectivity or, we might say, to one's being in the world in a much more *comprehensive* and *fundamental* manner. As Hagman suggests, this aspect of the feeling is based on the formalization of one's subjectivity *in toto* – that is, of having one's basic sense of being strengthened and reflected back to oneself in ideal form. This side of the feeling tends to foreground one's *own* goodness rather than the worthy or successful elements of the painting. To be sure, the two aspects of rightness go hand in hand in experience: as the artist basks in the glory of her work, she feels both herself *and* the painting to be valuable, perhaps even perfect.

In this chapter, I have also touched upon the developmental dynamics that presumably underlie later artistic feelings of rightness. In line with Townsend and Hagman, I maintain that we learn to realize – to make 'real' – elements of our inchoate experience in and through our earliest interactions with others. When our experiential states are ideally reflected and corroborated via these exchanges, we also experience rudimentary feelings of fittingness, harmony, and resonance. This, in turn, instills in us a permanent desire to engage with objects that feel right and make us feel right, too. In a gradual and crucial turn of events, we learn to *create* such objects for ourselves, first by adopting specific transitional objects and later by making art. As our experiencing steadily grows to be more sedimented and sophisticated, the objects we create for ourselves also become imbued with an increasing array of experiential elements. For this reason, we should avoid all simple reduction of mature feelings of rightness to significantly earlier ones.

To conclude, I submit that the need to 'get it right' reflects the perpetual existential concerns of being fully alive and meaningfully connected with the world. Simply put, we continuously seek relationships that affirm and enhance our being. To quote Winnicott, what we need and desire most is "to feel that life is real, to find life worth living" (Winnicott, 1971, p. 98). The feeling of getting one's painting right can go a long way in bringing about these valuable affective effects.

Chapter 7

Painting and existential feeling

Thus far, I have suggested that painting consists in the creation of a niche that scaffolds various special feelings. I have also submitted that painting is a creative form of object-relating that is partially rooted in early infant–caregiver interactions. Crucially, I have argued that these primary exchanges establish several existential concerns that continue to structure adult experience and behavior. I have specified four such concerns, namely, how to relate subjective and objective realities; how to demarcate between self and not-self; how to cope with separation and the need to connect with others; and how to achieve and strengthen the sense of being alive. Through in-depth analyses of feelings of connectedness, resonance, vitality, and fusion, I have highlighted how the specified existential concerns become episodically manifest in the painterly process.

In this chapter, I dig even deeper. I elaborate on the fact that, besides enabling and supporting various transient affective states, art-making can have a profound effect on the artist's overall sense of being. To support this claim, I provide a case study of psychoanalyst Marion Milner's (1957) intensive experimentation with painting. Milner, more acutely perhaps than any other psychoanalytic writer, reflected on the ways in which art-making relates to overall creative living. To expound further on her painterly project and its existential implications, I make use of philosopher Matthew Ratcliffe's (2008, 2015) theory of so-called existential feelings. Put broadly, existential feelings constitute a changeable background sense of what is real and possible, and as such, structure how we belong to and relate to the world as a whole. Within this conceptual framework, I argue that Milner's creative progression can be understood both as temporary shifts in existential feeling and as the gradual consolidation of a more permanent existential orientation. To conclude the chapter, I consider the wider applicability of Milner's case to the understanding of painterly affectivity. All in all, my aim is to show that painting, and especially a long-term commitment to painting, can significantly reconfigure how one finds oneself in the world.

Shifting realities in Milner's *On Not Being Able to Paint*

Milner arrived at her artistic exploration in a rather intriguing manner. After studying the effects of conventional education on schoolchildren for several years, she found herself increasingly drawn to what she called the problem of psychic creativity (Milner, 1957, p. xvii). To investigate the matter further, Milner decided to learn how to paint – a pastime that she had previously engaged in as a 'Sunday-painter', but with mostly disappointing results. In the literary output of her project, *On Not Being Able to Paint* (published originally in 1950), Milner provides a vivid self-observational description of her artistic journey, reflecting, for example, on her developing understanding of form, content, and color, and on the perceptual and affective aspects of her overall creative progression. Crucially, as her painterly endeavor unfolds, its existential reverberations rise to the fore and become established as pivotal elements in both art-making and creative living. In what follows, I review the main trajectory of Milner's creative enquiry and elaborate on its key findings.

What the eye likes: searching for the life of painting

At the outset of her efforts, Milner was mostly frustrated. Relying on received conventions of beauty, proportionality, and perspective had resulted in lifeless pictorial results. For Milner, such pictures embodied a mode of perception in which the world was "quite clearly and precisely 'there'", yet "remained utterly remote and meaningless" (1957, p. 21). Moreover, making accurate yet detached copies of reality had amounted to feelings of futility about the whole occupation of painting. Incidentally, similar sentiments have been a driving force for numerous more established painters as well, including Lucien Freud. As Martin Gayford writes,

> what he [Freud] was after was quite different: a picture that would have a life of its own. And that was not achieved by an artist who

> merely copied nature superficially, it was necessary to change it. What the picture should contain was the artist's own feelings and thoughts about the subject, put together in such a way that it acquired a power and presence of its own.
>
> (Gayford, 2018, p. 118)

To overcome her sense of paintings' insignificance and futility, Milner decided to pursue "what the eye really liked" (1957, pp. 3–4). Her primary method in this was to draw without predetermined depictive aims or preconceived notions of beauty and propriety. In and through these "free drawings", Milner discovered several important things. First, she found the drawings to express feelings and thoughts that were normally inhibited by the aim of making conventionally 'good' pictures. Moreover, the drawings sometimes appeared to be better-ordered wholes than those with clearly planned intent (pp. 4–8, 71). Second, she noted that achieving the vital expressivity characteristic of the free drawings called for a particular type of concentration: a "mood of reciprocity" in which eye and hand were free to respond spontaneously to the emerging marks on the paper (pp. 71–76). Finally, and most weightily, Milner recognized that the free drawings, or at least some of them, were "complicated reflections upon the central problems of being alive" (p. 74), the most pressing of these being how to bring one's imaginative capacities into creative interplay with the realities of the external world.

In addition to the free drawings, Milner experimented with the depiction of more fixed arrangements, compositions, and scenes – both imagined and perceived. In doing so, she realized that creating vital pictures required her to become much more "mixed up" with the objects of her painterly interests (1957, p. 10). Together with this immersed contemplation came an intense feeling for and belief in the living reality of the things observed. At its most striking, the approach led to

> a complete transfiguration of the common sense expedient view where objects, both people and things, existed mainly in terms of their usefulness; it brought a change to a world of living essences existing in their own right and offering a source of delight simply through the fact of being themselves.
>
> (p. 21)

In Milner's account, then, the habitual common-sense view of the world was rigidly utilitarian, reminiscent of the action mode of Deikman's model of bimodal consciousness, whereas the *transfigured view* made room for the receptive mode of attending to objects on their own terms (see Chapter 5). Milner notes that the latter way of perceiving left her "continually searching for its return", and also had her questioning whether it might in fact be "more real" than the common-sense mode of experiencing things (p. 21).

Another turning point for Milner was the revelation that, in concentrated looking, the *outlines* between perceived objects were not inherently clear cut. She describes, for example, how the edges between two jugs began to "ripple" in relation to one another (1957, p. 16). This sensation of indistinctness was reinforced by her perceptions of *color*. When colors were "freed from the bondage to natural appearance and outline", they moved and merged with each other much more fluidly than habitual perception permitted (p. 22). Seen like this, color had a living quality instead of being flatly fixed within the bounds of sharply demarcated entities.

Slowly but surely, then, Milner grew aware of two different experiential worlds: that of common sense, clear distinctions, and fixity – basically, a world in which things are separate and stay the same – and that of change, development, and fluid boundaries – a world where things continuously intermix and merge with each other. This disclosure was also somewhat unsettling, as it gave rise to a "dim fear" of losing one's hold on the solid ground of reality (1957, p. 16). Such apprehensiveness led Milner to believe that there were strong emotional forces working against the undoing of boundaries, if only even temporarily. On the other hand, surrendering to a more fluid mode of experience felt potentially liberating, and thus enticing. After reflecting on this tension, Milner surmised that the tendency to imprison objects within themselves served to tether the self to a presumably secure world of factual reality.

Eventually, Milner's incipient concern over boundaries gained special prominence in her discussion of creativity. It also took on various different forms. Informed at first by her fluid perceptions of *external objects*, she went on to conjecture that the *surrounding world as a whole* was in flux – that is, in a continuous process of change in which there is "no sharp line between one state and the next" (1957, p. 24). The gradual merging of one state into the other, she adds, seemed to reflect the "true quality of experience itself" (p. 24). In the context of this universal flux, Milner also considered the more specific issue of *self–other* boundaries:

> And this idea of there being no fixed outline, no boundary between one state and another, also introduced the idea of no boundary between one self and another self, it brought in the idea of one personality merging with another.
>
> (p. 24)

Finally, and perhaps most prominently, she called attention to "the boundaries between the tangible realities of the external world and the imaginative realities of the inner world of feeling and idea" (p. 17). Like Winnicott, Milner believed that the permeability of *internal-external* boundaries enabled the suffusion of objective reality with one's imagination and was therefore a precondition for vital creative living. Based on these reflections, Milner arrived at a momentous conclusion: "To be able to *break down* the barrier of space between self and other, yet at the same time to be able to *maintain* it, this seems to be the paradox of creativity" (p. 144, my italics).

All in all, we can see a major thread developing in Milner's painterly exploration: whether through free drawings, more traditional attempts at depiction, or simply by looking at things differently, a new reality was gradually making itself known to her. To open herself to this reality, Milner had to surrender the common-sense, detached way of looking, which in turn demanded "facing certain facts about oneself as a separate being, facts that could often perhaps be successfully by-passed in ordinary living" (1957, p. 13). Indeed, she soon found herself pondering the experiential constitution of spatial reality altogether: how feelings of distance, separation, having, losing, merging, and togetherness were grounded in being a body amongst other bodies in space. In the final analysis, Milner realized that these kinds of existential issues were the painter's "main preoccupation" (p. 12). Indeed, she concludes *On Not Being Able to Paint* with two chapters titled "Painting and living" and "Painting as making real" respectively. This clearly demonstrates that, by the time her project was drawing to a close, Milner had come to see painting as a thoroughly existential affair.

There are three key points that illuminate further Milner's understanding of the existential undercurrent of painting:

1 In basic psychoanalytic fashion, Milner acknowledged that the objective world possesses a reality that does not readily succumb to our subjective and often unconscious wishes, fantasies, and desires. This disillusioning fact – the realization of an irreversible subject–object split – could be a source of primitive hate, frustration, and despair. On the other hand, as Winnicott so painstakingly demonstrated, disillusionment is a developmental prerequisite for experiencing objects as having autonomous existence, that is, as being 'objectively real' (see Chapter 3). All individuals must therefore deal with the inevitable ramifications of a primary subject–object split. One of Milner's main conclusions was that artwork could be a *purposive means* to address this basic human concern. As she puts it: "It is surely through the arts that we deliberately restore the split and bring subject and object together into a particular kind of new unity" (1957, p. 131). In her view, art is an area of "vital illusion" in which we need not decide what is self and what is not, and by which we infuse reality with new life and significance (pp. 30, 138). Crucially, by accepting the necessity of *both* disillusion *and* illusion, primary hate/despair can be creatively transcended and permanently mitigated.

   In this connection, Milner also noted that art-making requires a *special type of labor*, "not in the way of the practical work of the world, but in an 'as if' way" (1957, p. 131). That is, in artwork a new subject–object unity is achieved through the purposeful manipulation of a malleable material. On the one hand, a chosen bit of the objective world is diligently yet playfully modified to fit subjective experience. On the other, the reshaped object remains a part of external reality – "it is still paint or stone or spoken or written words or movements of bodies or sounds of instruments" (p. 131). Upon completion, the work of art becomes a perceivable and shareable instantiation of the newly formed bond between the artist's imagination and the surrounding world. Seen in this way, the art object emerges and exists in a special 'as-if' area between internal and external realities or, to put it in explicitly Winnicottian terms, in the potential space wherein subjective and objective coincide in play.

2 Milner also recognized that painting is fundamentally concerned with *what one seeks to give*. Ideally, the artist will find a niche that needs what she has to offer – a "gap" into which she can pour her energies and in which she can feel that her offerings are wanted and appreciated (1957, p. 133). Whether or not this gap is found in actual social recognition depends on various fortuitous circumstances. Needless to say, the artist must always commence from and work within some set of historical-cultural conventions, even if she ends up subverting these to a significant degree. There is thus a fine balance to be struck between obscurity and communicability, between pursuing one's personal vision and making it sufficiently shareable with others. Alas, the artist might never find an appreciative or understanding audience for her work.

But, whatever the public perception of the artist's contributions, her art-making will still contain a basic element of self-sufficiency. As Milner puts it, artists have the ability to *create their own gap*; not only do they "make the size of the gap" to suit themselves, but they must also "choose what shall fill it" (p. 133). In this manner, the artist can address the problem of giving in a way that is not overly dependent on the receptiveness or demands of actual others. Milner also describes this as the artist's invention of a 'halfway house' between an imagined, idealized receiver and a real, external one. This intermediate recipient is more pliable and more under the artist's own control than the external (social) world, but also more fixed and stable than a "merely internal dream receiver" (p. 133). To restate this in terms of affective scaffolding, in painting the painter sets up for herself an environmental niche that supports both the creative process of give and take and the desired feeling of producing something good and valuable.

3 Finally, Milner came to champion the *transformative power* of art-making. Through her creative efforts she proclaimed to have discovered a *different sense of self* and a *new way of being* (1957, p. 142). This indicates that one's 'self' and one's 'being in the world' are intimately connected, and that artistic creativity can impact both simultaneously. Milner expresses this idea succinctly: "Ultimately then it is ourselves that the artist in us is trying to create; and if ourselves, then also the world, because one's view of the one interpenetrates with one's view of the other" (p. 136).

Importantly, Milner found that the artistic recreation of one's experiential world typically involved a feeling of *enrichment*. She explains the dynamics behind this feeling as follows:

> Since the object is thereafter endowed with a bit of the "me", one can no longer see it in quite the same way as before; and since the "me", the inner experience, has become enriched with a bit more of external reality, there is now *a closer relation between wishes and what can really exist* and so less cause for hate, less despair of ever finding anything that satisfies. In fact the aesthetic experience has modified the wish, moulded a bit of oneself into a new form by giving it a new object; and at the same time it has given a previously indifferent bit of the outside world a new emotional significance.
>
> (1957, pp. 131–132, my italics)

When the split between subjective and objective realities is creatively overcome in art, a more unified bond between the two is forged. This in turn enhances the artist's feelings of significance, value, and connectedness.

Milner was confident that her creativity-related discoveries held relevance beyond the immediate context of art-making. Rhetorically, she asks: "[W]as it not also possible that this different sense of self that grew out of creative concentration had bearings upon one's relation to the whole mass of other selves that one was in contact with?" (1957, pp. 142–143). Related to this, Milner acknowledged that, on the one hand, we undeniably exist and interact as separate bodily entities, and that believing otherwise would be delusional. But she also saw that "the boundaries of one's spiritual identity . . . do not have to remain identical with one's skin" (p. 143). That is to say, we connect with others (and the world) in ways that overcome our objectively perceived physical boundaries. For Milner, the transcendence of bodily separateness was especially pertinent in the social sphere – evidenced, for example, by the union that people achieve as they work together for a common purpose. She also found that,

> in order to "realise" other people, make them and their uniqueness fully real to oneself, one has in a sense to put oneself into the other, one has to temporarily undo that separation of self and other which one had so laboriously achieved.
>
> (pp. 143–144)

On these grounds, Milner envisioned a collective overcoming of the detached attitude that is so prevalent in common-sense human relating. Such an attitude only stultifies the interplay of subjective and objective realities and hence, creative (social) living, as well.

Let us pause here to take stock. At heart, Milner's case illustrates a far-reaching process of existential change. Through sustained and concentrated looking, drawing, and painting, her basic sense of reality shifted dramatically. On a more general level, Milner's project indicates that, in and through painting, artists can tap into and remold their overall sense of being vis-à-vis demarcation, separateness, connectedness, vitality, and so on. In short, by their chosen means of creative environmental manipulation, painters may actively broaden and reorganize their experiential worlds. But an important question still lingers: How, precisely, should we account for the *affective* nature of these kinds of existential changes? It is to this question that I now turn.

The affective nature of Milner's creative transformation

As Milner's case aptly demonstrates, painting involves a plenitude of feelings. The painter may feel apprehensive about making the first mark on the canvas; anxious about producing something unsatisfactory; frustrated by problems of color and composition; absorbed by the developing work at hand; delighted about creating something new and surprising; somber about surrendering the finished work of art; and, in the end, proud of her achievement. In contemporary philosophy of mind, these kinds of feelings are commonly classified as *emotions*. As specified in Chapter 1, emotions are episodic intentional affective states directed towards relatively specific objects in the world: things, the self, other persons, events, actions, or states of affairs. To reiterate, in this context the term 'intentionality' refers to the fact that mental states are *about* or *directed towards* some object or other, broadly conceived. In the aforementioned emotions, the common intentional object is the work of art during its various phases of development.

Sometimes, however, the intentional objects of our affective states are not as clearly specifiable. In other words, 'what they are about' or 'directed towards' is much more vague. Affective states that have relatively indefinite intentional objects are often classified as *moods*. The painter may, for instance, feel angry at everything and nothing in particular without being able to put a finger on what it is that is so infuriating. This lingering mood will likely affect the more specific emotions she undergoes during her work – condensing, perhaps, into feelings of frustration and aggression towards the painting at hand.

Finally, there are occurrent affects that track our ongoing bodily states and processes exclusively and are hence classified as *bodily feelings*. For example, after hours of demanding work, the painter may feel sore in the joints, tired in the eyes, and heavy in the legs. In somewhat strained technical terms, such feelings are characterized as being intentionally directed towards one's own body or part(s) of it. To sum up, emotions, moods, and bodily feelings can be classified as intentional affective states that are directed at specific objects, unspecific objects, or one's own body, respectively (for further discussion, see, e.g., Ben Ze'ev, 1997; Goldie, 2000; Prinz, 2004; Ratcliffe, 2008; Deonna & Teroni, 2012; Colombetti, 2014).

With the given distinctions in mind, let us revisit Milner's transformative affective experience. She describes how, whenever she was able to break free from the tedious and mechanistic copying of nature to create vital pictures, something else happened: the "process always seemed to be accompanied by *a feeling that the ordinary sense of self had temporarily disappeared*" (1957, p. 154, my italics). Milner specifies that this pronounced shift from ordinary consciousness consisted in feelings of "blankness", "no-differentiation", and "elation" (pp. 154–155). Notably, she affirms that the experience also disclosed an entirely new, harmonious, and unified way of being:

> It was the discovery that when painting something from nature there occurred, at least sometimes, *a fusion into a never-before-known wholeness*; not only were the object and oneself no longer felt to be separate, but neither were thought and sensation and feeling and action. All one's visual perceptions of colour, shape, texture, weight, as well as thought and memory, ideas about the object and action towards it, the movement of one's hand together with the feeling of delight in the "thusness" of the thing, they all seemed fused into a *wholeness of being* which was *different from anything else that had ever happened to me*.
>
> (Milner, 1957, p. 142, my italics)

So, what precisely is happening here? Can Milner's affective experience be adequately discussed in terms of bodily feeling, emotion, and/or mood, as they have been defined earlier? To address this problem, I next discuss the plausibility of each option in turn.

First, could the given 'wholeness of being' be a *bodily feeling*? As it happens, Milner elaborated at length on the fundamentally bodily nature of painting (1957, pp. 106–121). She describes peak creativity in terms of "enhanced bodily awareness" and as a "state of total body concentration" (pp. 107, 111). In such moments of absorbed perception and action, the "imaginative body" spreads out to envelop the object(s) of one's creative interests (p. 55). I understand Milner's 'spreading of the imaginative body' to be a basic form of empathy: a kind of 'feeling into' (*Einfühlung*) wherein one projects oneself into another body (or the environment). Crucially, Milner found a "startling change in the quality of experience itself when imagination was brought down to earth and made incarnate in the body, a sudden richness that was like the sun coming out over a world that had been all greyness" (p. 121). Viewed in this light, the described feeling of enriched wholeness could certainly be seen as a significant shift in one's bodily-constituted experience of the world. Even so, it should not be confused with 'bodily feeling' in the previously specified, restricted sense of the term, for it is clearly not a feeling of the condition of the *body exclusively* nor of a change therein – akin to a racing heart or the sudden appearance of goose bumps. Hence, the claim that the feeling takes as its intentional object the body, or parts of it, is too narrow in scope.

Second, we could try to make sense of Milner's affective experience in terms of *emotion*. Pursuing this option would in turn require us to identify a sufficiently specific object towards which the feeling is directed. Perhaps the foremost option in this case would be to submit that the intentional object of her feeling is the object of her immediate attention, namely, whatever it is that she is painting. But this doesn't seem quite right, either. Although Milner experienced wholeness *while* painting 'something' from nature, it would be counterintuitive and contrary to her description to suggest that she felt wholeness *specifically about* whatever that painted 'something' happened to be.

If the intentional object of Milner's feeling is not something specific in her surroundings, we might then be prompted to ask: Could her feeling instead be about her 'self'? Certainly, we have all kinds of self-referential emotions in which our selves, or aspects of our selves, are disclosed *to ourselves* in a certain affective light. For example, we may feel pity for or disappointed with ourselves. Perhaps Milner's affective state could therefore be characterized as a feeling of wholeness which, ultimately, concerns her own self. Although there is some truth to this alternative, I find it rather contrived and phenomenologically unsound as well. Even though her feeling undeniably concerns the self, I believe it does so in a much more profound manner than mere self-referential emotions allow for. Whereas the latter represent a particular intentional object *within* the world (namely, the self) in a relatively selective, evaluative, and focused light (for example, as pitiful, embarrassing, or praiseworthy), Milner's affective state appears to concern her *standing in the world* more comprehensively. Simply put, her feeling does not merely disclose the self or one of its features under a limited affective aspect; it discloses the world – *including* the self, its boundaries, and its relations to other objects – in a more all-encompassing manner.

Finally, if we regard Milner's affective state as the suggested kind of world-disclosing feeling, why not classify it simply as a *mood*? Seeing as moods are distinguishable from emotions due to their vague intentionality, we might argue that the 'world' is a sufficiently indistinct intentional object to warrant the classification of her feeling as a mood. I think this is a step in the right direction, but it, too, can only take us so far. This is because the sense in which the 'world' is disclosed in Milner's experience of wholeness differs from the sense in which it is present as an indefinite intentional object in commonplace moods. The 'world' in the presently examined sense is a world of practical engagement that we are always necessarily immersed in, rather than some abstract object of our feelings. Simply put, it is more than a mere semantic placeholder for the perceived lack of a sufficiently distinct object for the specified affective state. For this reason, I submit that Milner's feeling is not a mood in the conventional sense of the term. However, as I argue next, it can still be classified as a mood, albeit one that is more profound in kind.

In sum, I have sought to demonstrate the insufficiency of the common conceptions of 'bodily feeling', 'emotion', and 'mood' in accounting for Milner's affective transformation. As suggested, her own account indicates that what she experienced was a significant change in her overall sense of being rather than any feeling directed towards herself, the world, or any of its objects specifically. That is to say, Milner's transformative experience appears to have incorporated the body, the self, and the world in ways that established models of affective intentionality cannot quite grasp. An alternative conceptual approach is therefore in order.

Existential feeling

I submit that philosopher Matthew Ratcliffe's theory of *existential feelings* (2005, 2008, 2015; see also Saarinen, 2018) can go a long way in making sense of Milner's creative transformation. To support this view, I first provide an overview of the basic tenets of his theory. Then, equipped with the appropriate conceptual tools, I reinterpret Milner's overall experiential transformation as shifts in existential feeling and as the establishment of a new existential orientation.

Ratcliffe holds that feelings can be classified as existential in virtue of two shared characteristics. First, they are *pre*-intentional background feelings that structure experience as a whole (Ratcliffe, 2015, pp. 33–58). A key philosophical source for this notion is Martin Heidegger's (1927/1996) analysis of *Befindlichkeit* and *Stimmung*. *Befindlichkeit* means that we always already find ourselves in a world that matters to us in some way. Finding oneself in the world is in turn affectively constituted by one or another *Stimmung* or 'mood'. Simply put, we are always attuned to the world through our moods. In this Heideggerian sense, we do not *have* moods in the same way that we have emotions, desires, or beliefs towards objects within the world. Instead we find ourselves *in* moods that disclose the world to us in a pre-given, all-encompassing manner.

Ratcliffe accordingly emphasizes the fact that, in Heideggerian terms, 'world' is not an object of any particular intentional mental state. Rather, it is a backdrop against which we are able to adopt intentional mental states of whatever kind towards objects or states of affairs within the world (Ratcliffe, 2015, p. 19). Moreover, Ratcliffe maintains that experiencing things within the context of a pre-given world also implicates a sense of the possible. As he puts it, "to find oneself in a world is to have a sense of the various ways in which things might be encountered" (2015, p. 51). On this account, the world is fundamentally a *space of possibilities* in which moods constitute the *kinds* of possibility we are receptive to. For example, feeling fear towards any object in the world presupposes the sense that the world includes the possibility of threat or danger.

The second key characteristic of existential feelings is that they are *bodily* feelings (Ratcliffe, 2015, pp. 59–64; for a critical discussion, see

Saarinen, 2018). To specify the sense in which existential feelings are bodily, Ratcliffe distinguishes them conceptually from so-called *noematic* and *noetic* bodily feelings (pp. 83–84). Simply put, *noematic* bodily feelings are feelings *of* the body or parts of the body. These are the kinds of bodily feelings I have discussed earlier, namely, feelings that take the body as their primary intentional object, such as the feeling of one's own heartbeat. However, as Ratcliffe notes, we do not generally experience our bodies as sealed containers, with some feelings falling neatly on the inside and others on the outside. Thus, in addition to being a *felt* body, the body is also a *feeling* body: a medium for world-directed experience. In *noetic* bodily feelings, then, the body is *that through which* objects other than one's body are experienced. Although the body is not an explicit object of attention in such feelings, it still contributes to intentional affective experience through a kind of background awareness – for instance, when one's rapidly beating heart contributes to the frightening feel of a menacing situation.

To make more sense of this, let us consider, for example, the state of effortless flow while painting. In such moments the painter's attention will be directed, at least for the most part, towards the world rather than towards her body. More precisely, the painter's main focus will be on the *painting-in-progress*: on the mixing of colors, on the way the paint spreads over the canvas, on the emergence of form and composition, and so on. All the while, *background* bodily feelings of openness and alertness provide the situation with an overall sense of absorption and fluidity. In this way, noetic bodily feelings are incorporated into experiencing the painting as receptive and responsive to one's painterly gestures. In contrast to this, the painter may gradually become frustrated by a formal or material problem in the painting. In this case, when she shifts her attention to her body, she might find herself to feel weighed down, confined, and tired. And, when her attention is once again turned from her body toward the painting, the given bodily feelings will continue to contribute noetically to experiencing the painting as increasingly resistant and overbearing. In this situation the painter might seek some fresh air to clear her head, stretch her limbs to break the deadlock, or choose to do something else altogether.

Crucially, unlike noematic and noetic bodily feelings, existential feelings cannot be classified as intentional states directed towards anything (either one's body or things in one's surroundings). Instead, they provide the "overall context in which we have intentional states with noetic and noematic aspects" (Ratcliffe, 2012, p. 39, 2015, pp. 59, 83). To elaborate, Ratcliffe identifies kinesthesia, proprioceptive awareness, interoceptive awareness of visceral feelings, and tactile background feelings as some of the main bodily "ingredients" of existential feelings (2008, p. 123, 2015, pp. 59–64). These 'ingredients' interact with each other in a variety of ways to produce a diffuse yet unitary "body sense" that has its own distinct phenomenology (2008, pp. 123–124, 2010, p. 600). This means that existential feelings are not merely sub-personal or unconscious bodily states or dispositions. They are, instead, *integral* to ongoing experience. Even so, existential feelings are not usually felt *as* bodily. Rather, any given existential feeling simply "*is* the way in which one finds oneself in the world" (Ratcliffe, 2008, pp. 124, 129, emphasis in original).

Due to their pre-intentionality, existential feelings tend to elude conscious awareness and precise verbalization. In everyday talk, they are typically described in all-enveloping terms, for instance, as feelings of unfamiliarity, strangeness, being at home, being at one, and so on (Colombetti & Ratcliffe, 2012, p. 147). Moreover, in such descriptions, 'self', 'body', and 'world' tend to be interchangeable. Expressions such as 'I feel strange', 'my body feels strange', and 'the world feels strange' can refer to the same existential feeling, simply picking out one aspect of the self–body–world experiential continuum (p. 147).

Existential feelings tend to become consciously salient and available for reflection only when they undergo significant *shifts* or *disruptions*. A notable change in the feeling is accordingly felt as "a changed relationship to the world as a whole" (Ratcliffe, 2008, p. 124). When this happens, the previously taken-for-granted world can become conspicuous in its absence. For instance, in religious conversion experience, "a world that is drained of life . . . can be shaken up so as to reveal a different and perhaps wider space of possibility, something *more*, something *greater*" (p. 274, emphasis in original). The opposite happens in transitions into pathological states such as psychosis and depression, wherein the individual's experiential world is characterized by a loss of connection to other people and to shared reality. These examples illustrate the fact that "changes in the overall style of experience, in existential feeling, are shifts in the kinds of possibilities one is receptive to" (Ratcliffe, 2015, p. 51).

Compared to common moods and emotions, then, existential feelings can be said to structure experience in a far more *profound* manner. They delimit which intentional states are possible and intelligible to begin with, and in this way set the parameters for the kinds of experiences we are capable of having at all (Ratcliffe, 2010, p. 604; see also Ratcliffe, 2013, pp. 159–160, 2015, p. 130). To clarify what this means, consider an artist feeling passionate about her painting and enjoying it on a regular basis. Feeling such enthusiasm and joy towards the painterly activity presupposes that she already inhabits a world in which experiencing things as interesting and rewarding is an actual, felt possibility. This existential feeling cannot, however, be taken for granted. Someone who is deeply depressed will find herself in a world that is devoid of significance, vitality, and pleasurable activity. For her, everything feels fundamentally and inescapably lacking in delight and appeal. This is not a feeling directed *towards* a situation; it *is* the situation. Thus, enjoying painting ceases to be a real possibility.

In a nutshell, existential feelings are *feelings of being*: they constitute a changeable sense of reality and possibility, and of belonging to and relating to the world. With this concept now in use, I return one last time to Milner's artistically induced experiential transformation.

Painting an existential orientation

When Milner writes of her emergence into a new world of fluid boundaries, living essences, and wholeness, I maintain that she is describing a *significant change* in her underlying existential feeling. What she identifies as a 'shift from ordinary consciousness' quite evidently amounts to a new sense of reality or, to put it in phenomenological terms, to a new way of finding oneself in the world. It is revealing that Milner also discusses such moments in both self-related terms as the disappearance of an ordinary sense of self and in bodily terms as the spreading of the imaginative body. Taken together, her depictions aptly illustrate how self, body, and world are inextricably intertwined in existential feeling.

As shown, Milner's creative endeavor was frequently punctuated by notable changes in her habitual feeling of being. But there is more to her story than just temporary and seemingly arbitrary alterations in existential feeling. As Ratcliffe notes,

> when we reflect upon changes [in existential feeling], we come to recognize that there is a question to be addressed regarding the nature of

> our sense of reality, a question that cannot be asked if reality is taken as given.
>
> (Ratcliffe, 2008, p. 266)

This kind of reflection can provide us with insight into our lives as subjects – into what our lives amount to and what really matters to us. In short, notable shifts in existential feeling can open up our background orientations to a fundamental kind of self-interpretative evaluation (see Taylor, 1985, pp. 45–76). It is obvious that Milner reflected deeply on the existential perturbations and changes that she went through; indeed, I interpret *On Not Being Able to Paint* first and foremost as a record of these very deliberations. Having overcome her initial fears, Milner found the disruptions to her habitual sense of reality liberating and vitalizing, and hence, desirable. Crucially, they pushed her to question the world that she had previously inhabited and taken for granted.

Ultimately, Milner was captivated by the possibility of establishing an entirely new way of being (1957, p. 91). In her personal way she realized that, once our existential feelings became consciously salient, they could be significantly reshaped via various different activities, including artistic work. To put this in slightly different terms, transient episodic shifts in existential feeling can lead to the cultivation and consolidation of a new *existential orientation* – that is, a relatively stable and permanent way of finding oneself in the world. As outlined, Milner's transition from one orientation to another was based on her recognition of two modes of relating to the world: the common-sense mode of objective fact, and the imaginative mode of subjective fantasy, wish, and desire. Moreover, as Milner repeatedly points out, disillusionment – "the opening of one's eyes to what are called the stern facts of life" – meant recognizing that one's inner dream and outer reality could never completely and permanently coincide; they could only *interact* (1957, p. 89). For her, the critical existential concern was therefore how to achieve and maintain a *constructive interplay* between the two basic modes of experience.

By the end of her project, Milner had become fully aware that her artistically discovered existential orientation not only altered her private approach to art-making but also had wider social ramifications. Most importantly, it opened up alternative ways of connecting with others and generated new ideas for revising rigid educational practices. Echoing

Ratcliffe, we may thus conclude that Milner's newfound existential orientation disclosed to her a wider space of possibility – something more, something greater – and all of this was achieved through her dedicated experimentation with painting.

Concluding remarks

To conclude, I want to say a few words about the wider theoretical implications of Milner's case. To be sure, *On Not Being Able to Paint* does not purport to divulge any universal truths about artistic creativity or the practice of painting. Indeed, Milner was careful not to venture too far beyond personal experience in her descriptions and judgments of these processes. She spells out her position clearly:

> As for the validity of the ideas about what I was doing when painting, whether they held for other people and in other times and places I did not know. Probably not. Perhaps some people could paint without needing to have any clear idea about what they were doing and some found quite different ideas. Probably the particular idea that served to spark the creative process could vary widely and depended upon one's own particular experience and moment of existence in history.
>
> (Milner, 1957, p. 141)

Throughout this study, I have tried to adopt a similarly moderate and context-sensitive approach to analyzing painting and its affective nature. Hence, I have no interest in using Milner's case to generalize about what painting is, how it should be practiced, or what kinds of affective aims it should have.

That said, I do wish to extract from Milner's project one generally applicable idea, namely, that painting can have a profound effect on the artist's overall sense of being. Simply put, painting can serve to scaffold – to enable, support, regulate, and transform – the artist's existential feelings. It should moreover be noted that, although I have used Milner's case exclusively to spell out this claim, hers is by no means the only experiential account of artistic creativity that supports the proposed view. Michael Krausz, for example, describes his art-making illuminatively as follows:

> As a consequence of my nondualistic experience . . . I now experience more clearly, more expansively, more richly, more perspicuously.

> Such changes in my ways of experiencing in turn affect what I produce. What I produce has affected my ways of experiencing. I think of my art-making as a process in which who I am is enriched and transformed. In short, my art-production fosters my self-transformation, and my self-transformation fosters my art-production.
>
> (Krausz, 2009, p. 192)

This excerpt points to a tight and ongoing reciprocal relationship between Krausz's artwork and his overall way of experiencing the world.

In sum, painting does not only scaffold various episodic feelings but can also support the modification and sustenance of one's overall, affectively constituted existential orientation. Viewed in this light, existential feeling can become one of the main *objects* of artistic creativity – *that which is worked on* in painting. With varying degrees of conscious awareness, intent, and control, artists can tap into and reorganize their experiential worlds vis-à-vis demarcation, separateness, connectedness, vitality, and so on. George Hagman encapsulates this notion nicely when he suggests that "artistic creativity is not just something the artist does, a pastime or preoccupation, it is a way of being in the world and of experiencing one's inner and outer life". He continues: "Like breath or sight, the creative act is inseparable from self and, over time and effort, it becomes the artist's primary medium of self-experience, and self-in-relation to the world, and other people" (Hagman, 2010, p. 171). Indeed, when one commits one's entire life to painting, it may come to scaffold the most basic feeling of 'going on being', as Winnicott would put it. Embracing these core questions artistically and thus creating oneself and the world anew may well become the work of a lifetime.

Postscript

In this study, I have submitted a straightforward claim: that painters paint in order to feel. To explain how and why this is the case, I have, on the one hand, conceived of painting as a reciprocal form of affective scaffolding and, on the other hand, as an activity that incorporates some of the key relational needs and dynamics established in early environmental interaction. Moreover, I have systematically emphasized the existential significance of painting by tracing its connections to several core concerns that we must all perpetually deal with, and by exploring how painting enables painters to regulate and transform their fundamental feelings of being in the world. On the whole, I submit that these existential themes are already present in Winnicott's thinking, more or less explicitly; I have merely sought to pick them out and elaborate on them in the specific context of painting.

Without doubt, my account of affectivity in painting is limited in its range. I have focused mainly on feelings with generally positive valence and have thus left aside feelings that are more mixed, heavy, or downright negative. This has been a conscious decision informed by two key factors. First, it seems to me that much academic investigation into affectivity has tended to center on the negative, disturbing, and/or pathological. While inquiries into these types of feelings are highly interesting and relevant, and, moreover, hold significant clinical import, I have sought to bring some buoyancy to the given field of research. To that end, I have analyzed painting as a crucial means of vitalizing, enriching, and enhancing one's affective life. I have nonetheless tried to do so without promulgating a one-sided or overly rosy picture of painterly affectivity. Second, the concept of scaffolding is a particularly handy tool for highlighting the potentially positive aspects of our experiential lives, as it enables us to explore in detail the ways in which we actively manipulate our environments to suit us better and, more importantly, to achieve desirable and highly valued affective ends. In this sense, it is a concept that practically 'invites' and 'demands' us to concentrate on how our strivings for vital and meaningful being shape the niches that we inhabit.

Having said that, I think the concepts of 'affective scaffolding' and 'existential concern' could also be applied to investigate how painting supports processes of, for instance, reparation and mourning, or of coming to terms with deep shame and guilt. To put this in more general terms, it would be interesting to explore the ways in which painting enables the painter to undergo affective states and processes which fall, in terms of their valence, somewhere between distinctly positive and negative, and which may be beneficial for the individual to feel – even if this is at times exceedingly difficult or painful. In sum, I believe that extending the proposed approach to inspect various other existentially significant affects could prove to be quite fruitful.

Continuing with the topic of different kinds of feelings, the reader may have noticed that, apart from discussing Hagman's 'aesthetic resonance', I have not dealt with *aesthetic* emotions at all, or, more precisely, have not designated any of the examined affective states as aesthetic per se. This too has been a conscious decision, and again there are two main reasons behind it. First, the term 'aesthetic' is notoriously hard to pin down, and to have even provided a satisfactory summary of its conceptual history and relations to experiences of, for example, pleasure, beauty, awe, and sublimity would have required at least a whole separate chapter. Second, while the nature of aesthetic emotions may be an interesting question in itself, taking a stand on what such emotions consist in has not been necessary for the main argument of this study. I maintain that the examined feelings of aliveness, dissolution, fusion, connectedness, and rightness are completely intelligible without reference to anything 'aesthetic'. If it does not add anything relevant to the experiential description, we may just as well do without it. Of course, this does not entail that there are no such things as aesthetic emotions; nor does it rule out applying the notions of affective scaffolding and existential concern to feelings which are, in one sense or another, identifiable as 'aesthetic'.

Another restriction of this study has been its emphasis on *individual* artists' experience of their *own* paintings-in-progress. This choice has effectively sidelined the collective aspects of making and experiencing art. To be clear, I have not intended to neglect the fact that painting can be a joint effort, or that paintings are usually shared with others and may thus serve to scaffold their viewers' feelings, as well. There is a whole other side to the story in which finished paintings are sent out into the world, into a variety of affective niches – be they exhibition spaces, hospitals, hotels, schools, libraries, or private homes. In sum, the capacity of paintings to scaffold feelings does not dissipate once they leave the artist's studio, and it would certainly be interesting to investigate how, for example, religious art has served to scaffold affect – and particularly various feelings of being – diachronically over centuries and generations.

On the whole, the present study points towards novel and exciting paths of further theoretical inquiry. I believe that dissecting how the mind works and how affectivity is structured in the specific context of painting may reveal something relevant about the nature of mind and affectivity *more generally*. For example, in Chapter 2, I briefly bring up the contentious issue of extended affectivity. Proponents of the extended mind theory argue that the mind does not reside exclusively in the brain or within one's biological boundaries. Instead, under certain conditions, environmental resources/objects can be incorporated by the thinking and feeling subject with the result that these elements become constitutive components of the subject's mind, which has therefore become extended, as it were. From this perspective, it is not warranted to single out the neural constituents of the individual's occurrent feelings as their sufficient or exclusive basis.

I believe that scrutinizing painting in similar terms could contribute productively to ongoing debates over extended affectivity. Indeed, I have suggested in this study that painting can form a tightly integrated and reciprocal painter–painting feedback loop; however, I have refrained from claiming that this interaction instantiates extended affectivity proper. My analysis of robust scaffolding in painting could be pushed further to see whether it supports the extended affectivity thesis, and also to probe whether the view from painting could open up new ways of looking at the entire issue.

Viewed from an interdisciplinary perspective, this study also raises intriguing questions about the connections between relationally oriented psychoanalysis and those philosophical theories of mind that underline its situated, scaffolded, and possibly extended nature. By bringing Winnicott's developmental thinking into dialogue with the concepts of niche construction and scaffolding, I have already uncovered several pertinent similarities between the two approaches. Both lay stress on our own activeness in influencing how we come to think and feel. Even more crucially, both maintain that our experience of ourselves, others, and the world is fundamentally codetermined by the environment in which we are embedded. It is therefore quite futile to investigate the subject of experience as an isolated entity cut off from its multiple environmental relations. To put this even more plainly, there is arguably no 'proper' subjectivity or self to speak of separate from its object relations and environmental entanglements. This basic premise constitutes a solid bridge between the mentioned approaches – a theoretical structure along which key ideas can be transferred back and forth.

All in all, the connections drawn in this study between relational psychoanalysis and philosophy of mind and emotion amount to no more than a tentative sketch – a potential starting point for something richer and more refined. It would be immensely appealing and rewarding to develop a more systematic, detailed, and comprehensive analysis of the (potential) complementarity of the given approaches. On the one hand, the two could be examined jointly to emphasize and improve each other's understanding of the constitution and unfolding of our experiential lives. The primary aim would thus be to achieve a state of mutual benefit and enrichment. This is essentially what I have tried to do in this study. On the other hand, and much more ambitiously, we could seek to integrate the two into a new and unified theoretical approach to self and mind. This would, of course, be a massive undertaking. My hope is that this little study of affectivity in painting can serve as an illuminating and encouraging step in this direction.

Bibliography

Abram, J. (2007). *The Language of Winnicott: A Dictionary of Winnicott's Use of Words*. London: Karnac Books.

Ackermann, R. (2017). Rita Ackermann by Josh Smith. *BOMB Magazine*, 139. http://bombmagazine.org/article/0609313/rita-ackermann.

Adamson, L. B. & Frick, J. E. (2003). The Still Face: A History of a Shared Experimental Paradigm. *Infancy*, 4 (4), 451–473.

Andersen, M., Schjoedt, U., Nielbo, K. L., & Sørensen, J. (2014). Mystical Experience in the Lab. *Method and Theory in the Study of Religion*, 26, 217–245.

Anderson, D. R. & Hausman, C. R. (1992). The Role of Aesthetic Emotion in R. G. Collingwood's Conception of Creative Activity. *Journal of Aesthetics and Art Criticism*, 50 (4), 299–305.

Ataria, Y. (2014). Where Do We End and Where Does the World Begin? The Case of Insight Meditation. *Philosophical Psychology*, 28 (8), 1128–1146.

Ataria, Y., Dor-Ziderman, Y., & Berkovich-Ohana, A. (2015). How Does It Feel to Lack a Sense of Boundaries? A Case Study of a Long-Term Meditator. *Consciousness and Cognition*, 37, 133–147.

Ben-Ze'ev, A. (1997). The Affective Realm. *New Ideas in Psychology*, 15 (3), 247–259.

Betterton, R. (1996). *An Intimate Distance: Women, Artists and the Body*. New York: Routledge.

Bollas, C. (1987). *The Shadow of the Object: Psychoanalysis of the Unthought Known*. New York: Columbia University Press.

Bollas, C. (1999). *The Mystery of Things*. London and New York: Routledge.

Bollas, C. (2018). The Transformational Object. In G. Kohon (ed.), *British Psychoanalysis: New Perspectives in the Independent Tradition*, 88–103. London and New York: Routledge.

Clark, A. (1997). *Being There: Putting Brain, Body, and World Together Again*. Cambridge, MA: MIT Press.

Clark, A. (2006). Language, Embodiment, and the Cognitive Niche. *Trends in Cognitive Sciences*, 10 (8), 370–374.

Collingwood, R. G. (1938/1958). *The Principles of Art*. Oxford: Oxford University Press.

Colombetti, G. (2014). *The Feeling Body: Affective Science Meets the Enactive Mind*. Cambridge, MA and London: The MIT Press.

Colombetti, G. (2017a). Enactive Affectivity, Extended. *Topoi*, 36 (3), 445–455.
Colombetti, G. (2017b). The Embodied and Situated Nature of Moods. *Philosophia*, 45, 1437.
Colombetti, G. & Krueger, J. (2015). Scaffoldings of the Affective Mind. *Philosophical Psychology*, 28 (8), 1157–1176.
Colombetti, G. & Ratcliffe, M. (2012). Bodily Feeling in Depersonalization: A Phenomenological Account. *Emotion Review*, 4 (2), 145–150.
Colombetti, G. & Roberts, T. (2015). Extending the Extended Mind: The Case for Extended Affectivity. *Philosophical Studies*, 172, 1243–1263.
Comte-Sponville, A. (2008). *The Book of Atheist Spirituality*. London: Bantam Press.
Cork, R. (2015). *Face to Face: Interviews with Artists*. London: Tate Publishing.
Craig-Martin, M. (2015). *On Being an Artist*. London: Art/Books Publishing.
Danto, A. (1972). *Mysticism and Morality: Oriental Thought and Moral Philosophy*. New York: Basic Books.
Deikman, A. J. (1963). Experimental Meditation. *Journal of Nervous and Mental Disease*, 136, 329–343.
Deikman, A. J. (1966). Deautomatization and the Mystic Experience. *Psychiatry: Interpersonal and Biological Processes*, 29, 324–338.
Deikman, A. J. (1971). Bimodal Consciousness. *Archives of General Psychiatry*, 25, 481–489.
Deonna, J. A. & Teroni, F. (2012). *The Emotions: A Philosophical Introduction*. London and New York: Routledge.
Ehrenzweig, A. (1953). *The Psychoanalysis of Artistic Vision and Hearing: An Introduction to a Theory of Unconscious Perception*. London: Routledge and Kegan Paul.
Ehrenzweig, A. (1967). *The Hidden Order of Art: A Study in the Psychology of Perception*. London: Phoenix Press.
Eigen, M. (1983). Dual Union or Undifferentiation? A Critique of Marion Milner's View of the Sense of Psychic Creativeness. *International Review of Psycho-Analysis*, 10, 415–428.
Elkins, J. (2000). *What Painting Is*. London and New York: Routledge.
Epstein, M. (1990). Beyond the Oceanic Feeling: Psychoanalytic Study of Buddhist Meditation. *International Review of Psychoanalysis*, 17, 159–165.
Fauteux, K. (1994). *The Recovery of Self: Regression and Redemption in Religious Experience*. Mahwah, NJ: Paulist Press.
Fauteux, K. (1995). Beyond Unity: Religious Experience, Creativity, and Psychology. *Journal of Aesthetic Education*, 29 (2), 93–101.
Fonagy, P. & Target, M. (2003). *Psychoanalytic Theories: Perspectives from Developmental Psychology*. London and Philadelphia: Whurr Publishers.
Forman, R. K. C. (1998). What Does Mysticism Have to Teach Us about Consciousness? *Journal of Consciousness Studies*, 5 (2), 185–201.
Freud, S. (1910/2006). *Leonardo da Vinci: A Memory of His Childhood* (A. Tyson, trans.). London and New York: Routledge.
Freud, S. (1930/1961). Civilization and Its Discontents (J. Strachey, trans.). In J. Strachey (ed.), *The Standard Edition of the Complete Psychological Works of Sigmund Freud*, Vol. 21, 64–145. London: Hogarth Press and the Institute of Psycho-Analysis.
Fuchs, T. (2013). The Phenomenology of Affectivity. In K. W. M. Fulford, M. Davies, R. G. T. Gipps, G. Graham, J. Z. Sadler, G. Stanghellini, & T. Thornton (eds.), *The Oxford Handbook of Philosophy and Psychiatry*, 612–631. Oxford: Oxford University Press.

Fuchs, T. & De Jaegher, H. (2009). Enactive Intersubjectivity: Participatory Sense-Making and Mutual Incorporation. *Phenomenology and the Cognitive Sciences*, 8, 465–486.

Fuller, P. (1980). *Art and Psychoanalysis*. London: Writers and Readers Publishing Cooperative.

Gayford, M. (2018). *Modernists & Mavericks: Bacon, Freud, Hockney & the London Painters*. London: Thames and Hudson.

Geels, A. (1982). Mystical Experience and the Emergence of Creativity. *Scripta Instituti Donneriani Aboensis*, 11, 27–62.

Goldie, P. (2000). *The Emotions: A Philosophical Exploration*. Oxford: Oxford University Press.

Goldie, P. (2008). Freud and the Oceanic Feeling. In W. Lemmens & W. Van Herck (eds.), *Religious Emotions: Some Philosophical Explorations*, 219–229. Cambridge: Cambridge Scholars Publishing.

Graham, G. (2005). *Philosophy of the Arts: An Introduction to Aesthetics*. London and New York: Routledge.

Graw, I. (2018). *The Love of Painting: Genealogy of a Success Medium* (B. Hanrahan & G. Jackson, trans.). Berlin: Sternberg Press.

Griffiths, P. E. & Scarantino, A. (2009). Emotions in the Wild. In P. Robbins & M. Aydede (eds.), *The Cambridge Handbook of Situated Cognition*, 437–453. Cambridge: Cambridge University Press.

Gruen, J. (1991). *The Artist Observed: 28 Interviews with Contemporary Artists*. Chicago: A Cappella Books and Chicago Review Press.

Hagman, G. (2005). *Aesthetic Experience: Beauty, Creativity, and the Search for the Ideal*. Amsterdam: Rodopi.

Hagman, G. (2010). *The Artist's Mind: A Psychoanalytic Perspective on Creativity, Modern Art and Modern Artists*. London: Routledge.

Harrison, I. B. (1986). On "Merging" and the Fantasy of Merging. *The Psychoanalytical Study of the Child*, 41, 155–170.

Heersmink, R. & Sutton, J. (2018). Cognition and the Web: Extended, Transactive, or Scaffolded? *Erkenntnis*. Online first: https://doi.org/10.1007/s10670-018-0022.

Heidegger, M. (1927/1996). *Being and Time (Sein und Zeit)* (J. Stambaugh, trans.). New York: SUNY.

Horner, T. M. (1985). The Psychic Life of the Young Infant: Review and Critique of the Psychoanalytic Concepts of Symbiosis and Infantile Omnipotence. *American Journal of Orthopsychiatry*, 55 (3), 324–344.

Huttula, K. (2017). Värien vanki: Psykoterapeutti-taiteilija Maisa Kelan haastattelu. *Psykoanalyyttinen psykoterapia*, 13, 160–165.

Jäämeri, H. (2007). Kohtaan taulun kuin henkilön. *Suomen Kuvalehti*, 41. http://suomenkuvalehti.fi/jutut/kulttuuri/kohtaan-taulun-kuin-henkilon.

Khatchadourian, H. (1965). The Expression Theory of Art: A Critical Evaluation. *The Journal of Aesthetics and Art Criticism*, 23 (3), 335–352.

Koestler, A. (1954). *The Invisible Writing*. New York: The MacMillan Company.

Koestler, A. (2009). The Three Domains of Creativity. In M. Krausz, D. Dutton, & K. Bardsley (eds.), *Philosophy of History and Culture, Vol. 28: The Idea of Creativity*, 251–266. Boston: Brill.

Kohut, H. (2011). *The Search for the Self: Selected Writings of Heinz Kohut: 1950–1978* (P. H. Ornstein, ed.). London: Karnac.

Kovel, J. (1990). Beyond the Future of an Illusion: Further Reflections on Freud and Religion. *The Psychoanalytic Review*, 77 (1), 69–87.

Krausz, M. (2009). Creativity and Self-Transformation. In M. Krausz, D. Dutton, & K. Bardsley (eds.), *Philosophy of History and Culture, Vol. 28: The Idea of Creativity*, 191–203. Boston: Brill.

Kris, E. (1952). *Psychoanalytic Explorations in Art*. New York: International Universities Press.

Krueger, J. (2014a). Emotions and the Social Niche. In C. von Scheve & M. Salmela (eds.), *Collective Emotions*, 156–171. Oxford: Oxford University Press.

Krueger, J. (2014b). Varieties of Extended Emotions. *Phenomenology and the Cognitive Sciences*, 13 (4), 533–555.

Krueger, J. (2018). Schizophrenia and the Scaffolded Self. *Topoi*. Online first: https://doi.org/10.1007/s11245-018-9547-3.

Krueger, J. (forthcoming). Music as Affective Scaffolding. In D. Clarke, R. Herbert, & E. Clarke (eds.), *Music and Consciousness II*. Oxford: Oxford University Press.

Krueger, J. & Szanto, T. (2016). Extended Emotions. *Philosophy Compass*, 11 (12), 863–878.

Lachmann, F. M. & Beebe, B. (1989). Oneness Fantasies Revisited. *Psychoanalytic Psychology*, 6 (2), 137–149.

Laland, K., Matthews, B., & Feldman, M. W. (2016). An Introduction to Niche Construction Theory. *Evolutionary Ecology*, 30 (2), 191–202.

Levin, D. M. (1988). *The Opening of Vision: Nihilism and the Postmodern Situation*. New York: Routledge.

Lindahl, J. R. & Britton, W. B. (2019). "I Have This Feeling of Not Really Being Here": Buddhist Meditation and Changes in Sense of Self. *Journal of Consciousness Studies*, 26 (7–8), 157–183.

Loewald, H. (2000). *The Essential Loewald: Collected Papers and Monographs*. Hagerstown, MD: University Publishing Group.

Lynch, D. (2006). *Catching the Big Fish: Meditation, Consciousness, and Creativity*. New York: Tarcher and Penguin.

Maclagan, D. (2001). *Psychological Aesthetics: Painting, Feeling and Making Sense*. London: Jessica Kingsley Publishers.

Maharaj, A. (2017). The Challenge of the Oceanic Feeling: Romain Rolland's Mystical Critique of Psychoanalysis and His Call for a 'New Science of the Mind'. *History of European Ideas*, 43 (5), 474–493.

Mahler, M., Pine, F., & Bergman, A. (1989). *The Psychological Birth of the Infant: Symbiosis and Individuation*. London: Karnac.

Maiese, M. (2016). Affective Scaffolds, Expressive Arts, and Cognition. *Frontiers in Psychology*, 7, 359.

Masson, J. M. (1980). *The Oceanic Feeling: The Origins of Religious Sentiment in India*. Dordrecht: Reidel.

Matravers, D. (2010). Expression in the Arts. In P. Goldie (ed.), *The Oxford Handbook of Philosophy of Emotion*, 617–634. Oxford: Oxford University Press.

Meissner, W. W. (2005). On Putting a Cloud in a Bottle: Psychoanalytic Perspectives on Mysticism. *Psychoanalytic Quarterly*, 74 (2), 507–559.

Merkur, D. (1999). *Mystical Moments and Unitive Thinking*. New York: SUNY.

Millière, R., Carhart-Harris, R. L., Roseman, L., Trautwein, F.-M., & Berkovich-Ohana, A. (2018). Psychedelics, Meditation, and Self-Consciousness. *Frontiers in Psychology*, 9, 1475.

Mills, J. (1999). The Ontology of Religiosity: The Oceanic Feeling and the Value of the Lived Experience. *Religious Humanism*, 33 (3/4), 20–41.

Milner, M. (1950/1957). *On Not Being Able to Paint*. New York: Tarcher and Putnam.

Milner, M. (1987). *The Suppressed Madness of Sane Men: Forty-Four Years of Exploring Psychoanalysis*. London: Tavistock.

Nahm, M. C. (1955). The Philosophy of Aesthetic Expression. *The Journal of Aesthetics and Art Criticism*, 13 (4), 458–468.

Nelson, B. & Rawlings, D. (2007). Its Own Reward: A Phenomenological Study of Artistic Creativity. *Journal of Phenomenological Psychology*, 38, 217–255.

Newton, S. (2001). *Painting, Psychoanalysis, and Spirituality*. Cambridge: Cambridge University Press.

Newton, S. (2008). *Art and Ritual: A Painter's Journey*. London: Ziggurat.

Nielsen, J., Kruger, T. H. C., Hartmann, U., Passie, T., Fehr, T., & Zedler, M. (2013). Synaesthesia and Sexuality: The Influence of Synaesthetic Perceptions on Sexual Experience. *Frontiers in Psychology*, 4, 751.

Odling-Smee, F. J., Laland, K. N., & Feldman, M. W. (2003). *Niche Construction: The Neglected Process in Evolution*. Princeton, NJ: Princeton University Press.

Ostow, M. (2007). *Spirit, Mind, & Brain: A Psychoanalytic Examination of Spirituality & Religion*. New York: Columbia University Press.

Parsons, W. B. (1999). *The Enigma of the Oceanic Feeling. Revisioning the Psychoanalytic Theory of Mysticism*. Oxford: Oxford University Press.

Paul, E. S. & Kaufman, S. B. (2014). *The Philosophy of Creativity: New Essays*. Oxford: Oxford University Press.

Peterfreund, E. (1978). Some Critical Comments on Psychoanalytic Conceptualization of Infancy. *International Journal of Psychoanalysis*, 59, 427–441.

Pine, F. (2004). Mahler's Concepts of "Symbiosis" and Separation-Individuation: Revisited, Reevaluated, Refined. *Journal of the American Psychoanalytic Association*, 52, 511–533.

Prinz, J. (2004). *Gut Reactions: A Perceptual Theory of Emotion*. Oxford: Oxford University Press.

Ratcliffe, M. (2005). The Feeling of Being. *Journal of Consciousness Studies*, 12 (8–10), 43–60.

Ratcliffe, M. (2008). *Feelings of Being. Phenomenology, Psychiatry and the Sense of Reality*. Oxford: Oxford University Press.

Ratcliffe, M. (2010). Depression, Guilt and Emotional Depth. *Inquiry*, 53 (6), 602–626.

Ratcliffe, M. (2012). The Phenomenology of Existential Feeling. In S. Marienberg & J. Fingerhut (eds.), *Feelings of Being Alive*, 23–54. Berlin: de Gruyter.

Ratcliffe, M. (2013). Why Mood Matters. In M. A. Wrathall (ed.), *The Cambridge Companion to Heidegger's Being and Time*, 157–176. New York: Cambridge University Press.

Ratcliffe, M. (2015). *Experiences of Depression: A Study in Phenomenology*. Oxford: Oxford University Press.

Reddy, V. (2008). *How Infants Know Minds*. Cambridge, MA: Harvard University Press.

Rochat, P. (2003). Five Levels of Self-Awareness as They Unfold in Early Life. *Consciousness and Cognition*, 12, 717–731.

Rodman, F. R. (ed.). (1987). *The Spontaneous Gesture: Selected Letters of D. W. Winnicott*. Cambridge, MA: Harvard University Press.

Rolland, R. (1930/2009). *The Life of Vivekananda and the Universal Gospel* (25th ed., E. F. Malcolm-Smith, trans.). Kolkata: Swami Bodhasarananda.

Rooney, C. (2007). What Is the Oceanic? *Angelaki: Journal of the Theoretical Humanities*, 12 (2), 19–32.
Rose, G. (1980). *The Power of Form: A Psychoanalytic Approach to Aesthetic Form*. New York: International Universities Press.
Rotenberg, C. (1988). Selfobject Theory and the Artistic Process. *Progress in Self Psychology*, 4, 193–213.
Saarinen, J. A. (2012a). The Oceanic State: A Conceptual Elucidation in Terms of Modal Contact. *International Journal of Psychoanalysis*, 93 (4), 939–961.
Saarinen, J. A. (2012b). Teoreettisia lähtökohtia psykoanalyyttiseen taiteentutkimukseen. In A. Waenerberg & S. Kähkönen (eds.), *Taidetta tutkimaan – menetelmiä ja näkökulmia*, 259–279. Jyväskylä, Finland: Kampus Kustannus.
Saarinen, J. A. (2014a). The Oceanic Feeling: A Case Study in Existential Feeling. *Journal of Consciousness Studies*, 21 (5–6), 196–217.
Saarinen, J. A. (2014b). The Oceanic Feeling in Painterly Creativity. *Contemporary Aesthetics*, 12. www.contempaesthetics.org/newvolume/pages/article.php?articleID=704.
Saarinen, J. A. (2018). A Critical Examination of Existential Feeling. *Phenomenology and the Cognitive Sciences*, 17 (2), 363–374.
Saarinen, J. A. (2019). Paintings as Solid Affective Scaffolds. *The Journal of Aesthetics and Art Criticism*, 77 (1), 67–77.
Saarinen, J. A. (forthcoming). What Can the Concept of Affective Scaffolding Do for Us? *Philosophical Psychology*.
Sayers, J. (2007). *Freud's Art: Psychoanalysis Retold*. London and New York: Routledge.
Schwabsky, B. (2012). Conversation with Suzanne McClelland. *BOMB Magazine*, 118. https://bombmagazine.org/articles/suzanne-mcclelland/.
Silverman, D. (2004). Early Developmental Issues Reconsidered: Commentary on Pine's Ideas on Symbiosis. *Journal of the American Psychoanalytic Association*, 53, 239–251.
Slaby, J. (2014). Emotions and the Extended Mind. In C. von Scheve & M. Salmela (eds.), *Collective Emotions*, 32–46. Oxford: Oxford University Press.
Slaby, J. (2016). Mind Invasion: Situated Affectivity and the Corporate Life Hack. *Frontiers in Psychology*, 7, 266.
Spitz, E. H. (1985). *Art and Psyche: A Study in Psychoanalysis and Aesthetics*. New Haven, CT: Yale University Press.
Stephan, A., Walter, S., & Wilutzky, W. (2014). Emotions Beyond Brain and Body. *Philosophical Psychology*, 27, 65–81.
Sterelny, K. (2010). Minds: Extended or Scaffolded? *Phenomenology and the Cognitive Sciences*, 9 (4), 465–481.
Stern, D. N. (1985). *The Interpersonal World of the Infant: A View from Psychoanalysis and Developmental Psychology*. New York: Basic Books.
Stokes, A. (1955). *Michelangelo: A Study in the Nature of Art*. London: Tavistock.
Stokes, A. (1978). *The Critical Writings of Adrian Stokes, vol. III: 1955–1967*. London: Thames and Hudson.
Storr, A. (1989). *Solitude*. London: Harper Collins.
Stotz, K. (2010). Human Nature and Cognitive-Developmental Niche Construction. *Phenomenology and the Cognitive Sciences*, 9 (4), 483–501.
Stotz, K. (2017). Why Developmental Niche Construction Is Not Selective Niche Construction: And Why It Matters. *Interface Focus*, 7, 20160157.
Sutton, J. (2016). Scaffolding Memory: Themes, Taxonomies, Puzzles. In C. Stone & L. Bietti (eds.), *Contextualizing Human Memory: An Interdisciplinary Approach to*

Understanding How Individuals and Groups Remember the Past, 187–205. London and New York: Routledge.

Sutton, J., Harris, C. B., Keil, P. G., & Barnier, A. J. (2010). The Psychology of Memory, Extended Cognition, and Socially Distributed Remembering. *Phenomenology and the Cognitive Sciences*, 9 (4), 521–560.

Taipale, J. (2014). Facts and Fantasies: Embodiment and the Early Formation of Selfhood. In R. T. Jensen & D. Moran (eds.), *The Phenomenology of Embodied Subjectivity*, 241–262. London: Springer.

Taipale, J. (2016). Self-Regulation and Beyond: Affect Regulation and the Infant-Caregiver Dyad. *Frontiers in Psychology*, 7, 889.

Taylor, C. (1985). *Human Agency and Language: Philosophical Papers I.* Cambridge: Cambridge University Press.

Townsend, P. (2019). *Creative States of Mind: Psychoanalysis and the Artist's Process.* London and New York: Routledge.

Tronick, E. Z. (2003). Things Still to Be Done on the Still-Face Effect. *Infancy*, 4 (4), 475–482.

Tuymans, L. (2005). Conversation with Kerry James Marshall. *BOMB Magazine*, 92. http://bombmagazine.org/article/2733/luc-tuymans-and-kerry-james-marshall.

Varga, S. & Krueger, J. (2013). Background Emotions, Proximity and Distributed Emotion Regulation. *Review of Philosophy and Psychology*, 4, 271–292.

Vollenweider, F. X. (2001). Brain Mechanisms of Hallucinogens and Entactogens. *Dialogues in Clinical Neuroscience*, 3 (4), 266–279.

Vollenweider, F. X., Gamma, A., & Vollenweider-Scherpenhuyzen, M. F. I. (1999). Neural Correlates of Hallucinogen-Induced Altered States of Consciousness. In S. R. Hameroff, A. W. Kaszniak, & D. J. Chalmers (eds.), *Toward a Science of Consciousness III: The Third Tucson Discussions and Debates*, 99–110. Cambridge, MA: MIT Press.

Weber, B. (2018). Life. In Zalta, E. N. (ed.), *The Stanford Encyclopedia of Philosophy* (Summer 2018 ed). https://plato.stanford.edu/archives/sum2018/entries/life/.

Wentworth, N. (2005). *The Phenomenology of Painting*. Cambridge: Cambridge University Press.

Werman, D. (1986). On the Nature of the Oceanic Experience. *Journal of the American Psychoanalytical Association*, 34, 123–139.

Wilson, R. & Clark, A. (2009). How to Situate Cognition: Letting Nature Take Its Course. In P. Robbins & M. Aydede (eds.), *The Cambridge Handbook of Situated Cognition*, 55–77. Cambridge: Cambridge University Press.

Wiltsher, N. (2017). Feeling, Emotion, and Imagination: In Defence of Collingwood's Expression Theory of Art. *British Journal for the History of Philosophy*, 26 (4), 759–781.

Winnicott, D. W. (1953). Transitional Objects and Transitional Phenomena. *International Journal of Psychoanalysis*, 34 (2), 89–97.

Winnicott, D. W. (1965/2006). *The Family and Individual Development*. London and New York: Routledge.

Winnicott, D. W. (1971). *Playing and Reality*. London and New York: Routledge.

Wolson, P. (1995). The Vital Role of Adaptive Grandiosity in Artistic Creativity. *The Psychoanalytic Review*, 82 (4), 577–597.

Wright, E. (1998). *Psychoanalytic Criticism. A Reappraisal*. Cambridge: Polity Press.

Wright, K. (2009). *Mirroring and Attunement: Self-Realization in Psychoanalysis and Art.* London and New York: Routledge.

Index

For Product Safety Concerns and Information please contact our EU
representative GPSR@taylorandfrancis.com
Taylor & Francis Verlag GmbH, Kaufingerstraße 24, 80331 München, Germany

www.ingramcontent.com/pod-product-compliance
Ingram Content Group UK Ltd.
Pitfield, Milton Keynes, MK11 3LW, UK
UKHW011017180926
475701UK00004B/802

* 9 7 8 0 3 6 7 5 2 2 4 7 6 *